Mana 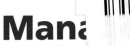 f the

BRITISH MENOPAUSE SOCIETY
Meeting the Challenge of Menopause

The ROYAL
SOCIETY *of*
MEDICINE
PRESS *Limited*

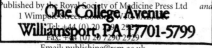

© 2006 Royal Society of Medicine Press Ltd and British Menopause Society Publications Ltd

Published by the Royal Society of Medicine Press Ltd   and   British Menopause Society Publications Ltd
1 Wimpole Street, London W1G 0AE, UK   4–6 Eton Place, Marlow, SL7 2QA, UK
Tel: +44 (0) 20 7290 2921   Tel: +44 (0) 1628 890199
Fax: +44 (0) 20 7290 2929   Fax: +44 (0) 1628 474024
Email: publishing@rsm.ac.uk   Email: admin.bms@btconnect.com
Website: www.rsmpress.co.uk   Website: www.the-bms.org

British Menopause Society (registered charity no. 10151440)

British Library Cataloguing in Publication Data
A catalogue record for this book is available from the British Library
ISBN 1 85315 667 1

Distribution in Europe and Rest of World:
Marston Book Services Ltd
PO Box 269
Abingdon
Oxon OX14 4YN, UK
Tel: +44 (0) 1235 465500
Fax: +44 (0) 1235 465555
Email: direct.order@marston.co.uk

Distribution in the USA and Canada:
Royal Society of Medicine Press Ltd
c/o BookMasters, Inc.
30 Amberwood Parkway
Ashland, Ohio 44805, USA
Tel: +1 800 247 6553 / +1 800 266 5564
Email: order@bookmasters.com

Distribution in Australia and New Zealand:
Elsevier Australia
30–52 Smidmore Street
Marrickville NSW 2204
Australia
Tel: + 61 2 9349 5811
Fax: + 61 2 9349 5911
Email: service@elsevier.com.au

Designed and typeset by Phoenix Photosetting, Chatham, Kent
Printed and bound by Krips b.v., Meppel, The Netherlands

Contents

About the editors

Margaret Rees is a Medical Gynaecologist and Reader in Reproductive Medicine in the Nuffield Department of Obstetrics and Gynaecology, University of Oxford. She runs the menopause clinic in Oxford – one of the first founded in the UK. She is Editor-in-Chief of the *Journal of the British Menopause Society*, and an expert advisor to Women's Health Concern.

David Purdie is Consultant to the Edinburgh Osteoporosis Centre and has a long clinical and research interest in the detection and treatment of osteoporosis. He is a former Chairman of Council of the British Menopause Society and a member of the scientific advisory group of the National Osteoporosis Society.

Preface

With the lifespan of women continuing to increase, and with many now surviving well into their 10th decade, the menopause can now be considered to be a mid-life event. Thus the problems of post-reproductive health are becoming key issues for health professionals. Publication of large randomized trials and observational studies in specific populations and the reactions to these by the media have generated confusion in both lay and professional circles about the best course to take.

The aim of the book is to provide a practical, unbiased and non-promotional guide for health professionals dealing with menopausal and postmenopausal women. The evidence base, where available, is presented. This fourth edition has been substantially revised and updated from the third, published in 2002. Previous editions have been cited by other organizations such as the Council of Affiliated Menopause Societies and form the template for menopause training modules for health professionals.

The book is in four sections: the menopause and postmenopausal health; assessment and investigations; management strategies; and women with special needs (such as those with a premature menopause). The design of clinical trials and practical methods of explaining risk are described. With regard to management strategies, both oestrogen and non-oestrogen-based treatments and their relative merits are discussed, as well as the evidence regarding alternative and complementary therapies.

This book has been the product of the activities of the Council of the British Menopause Society. Founded in 1989, the British Menopause Society aims to increase the awareness of post-reproductive health through specialist meetings and its publications, including its peer-reviewed and Medline-listed journal, *Journal of the British Menopause Society*. Other experts in the field have been consulted where required. We would like to thank the following for their contribution and comment:

Roger A'hern, London
Farook Al-Azzawi, Leicester
Gilly Andrews, London
Julie Ayres, Leeds
David Barlow, Glasgow
Heather Currie, Dumfries
Sarah Gray, Truro
Tim Hillard, Poole

Jean Hodson, Stratford-upon-Avon
Mary Ann Lumsden, Glasgow
Anthony Mander, Oldham
Jo Marsden, London
Lars-Ake Mattson, Goteborg, Sweden
Brigid McKevith, London
Martin Oehler, Melbourne, Australia

Nick Panay, London
Angela Panteli, Manchester
Anthony Parsons, Rugby
Joan Pitkin, Harrow
Bhanu Ruparelia, Worcester
John Stevenson, London

John Studd, London
David Sturdee, Solihull
Margaret Upsdell, Liverpool
Sovra Whitcroft, Guildford
Malcolm Whitehead, London
Jenny Williamson, Birmingham

Margaret Rees
David W Purdie
January 2006

THE MENOPAUSE AND POSTMENOPAUSAL HEALTH

1 The menopause: physiology and definitions

Introduction
Definitions
Stages of reproductive ageing
Ovarian function
Further reading

Introduction

The menopause is defined as the cessation of the menstrual cycle and is caused by ovarian failure. The term is derived from the Greek *menos*, meaning month, and *pausos*, meaning an ending. The median age at which the menopause occurs is 52 years. The age at menopause may be determined *in utero*, as growth restriction in late gestation, low weight gain in infancy and starvation in early childhood may be associated with an earlier menopause. It also occurs earlier in women with Down's syndrome and in smokers. Japanese race and ethnicity may be associated with later age of natural menopause.

A woman's average life expectancy at birth in the UK is currently 81 years; it is increasing and is estimated to reach 85 years by 2031. British women thus can expect more than 30 years of postmenopausal life, and, because more women will live to the age of 100 years, the menopause can now be considered to be a mid-life event.

Worldwide, increasing life expectancy and decreasing fertility rates mean that the number of people older than 65 years is projected to grow considerably in absolute and relative terms. In 2002, 440 million people were older than 65 years; this was about 7% of the total population. This figure is projected to increase rapidly, and it is estimated that the elderly will comprise nearly 17% of the world's population in 2050. The percentage of elderly people in the total population varies between countries, ranging from a high of 22% in Monaco to a low of 1.7% in Mayotte – an island in the Mozambique Channel. The percentage of elderly people is higher in the countries that make up the developed world and very low in Africa and the Near East.

In the UK the population is projected to increase by 7.2 million over the period 2004 to 2031 and will continue to rise thereafter until 2074, which is the end of the 2005 projections (Figure 1.1). From 2007 the population of state pensionable age will exceed the number of children and by 2031 is projected to exceed it by almost 4 million (34%).

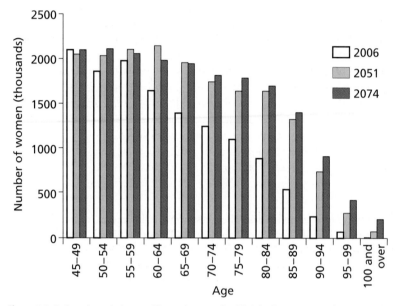

Figure 1.1 Projected population at mid-years by age at last birthday for women aged over 45 in the UK (thousands). Adapted from the Office of National Statistics and Government Actuaries Department (2005)

Definitions

Various definitions are in use and are detailed below.

- **Menopause** is the permanent cessation of menstruation that results from loss of ovarian follicular activity. Natural menopause is recognized to have occurred after 12 consecutive months of amenorrhoea for which no other obvious pathological or physiological cause is present. Menopause occurs with the final menstrual period and is thus known with certainty only in retrospect one year after the event. No adequate biological marker exists.
- **Perimenopause** includes the period beginning with the first clinical, biological and endocrinological features of the approaching menopause, such as vasomotor symptoms and menstrual irregularity, and ends 12 months after the last menstrual period.

- **Premenopause** is a term often used ambiguously to refer to the 1–2 years immediately before the menopause or to the whole of the reproductive period before the menopause. Currently, this term is recommended to be used in the latter sense, encompassing the entire reproductive period from menarche to the final menstrual period.
- **Postmenopause** should be defined from the final menstrual period regardless of whether the menopause was induced or spontaneous. Surgical menopause is timed precisely, but, as noted above, the time of natural menopause can only be determined retrospectively after a period of 12 months of spontaneous amenorrhoea.
- **Menopausal transition** is the period of time before the final menstrual period, when variability in the menstrual cycle is usually increased.
- **Climacteric** is the phase encompassing the transition from the reproductive state to the non-reproductive state. The menopause itself is thus a specific event that occurs during the climacteric – just as the menarche is a specific event that occurs during puberty.
- **Climacteric syndrome** – the climacteric is sometimes but not always associated with symptoms. When this occurs, the term 'climacteric syndrome' may be used.
- **Induced menopause** is the cessation of menstruation that follows surgical removal of both ovaries or iatrogenic ablation of ovarian function by chemotherapy, radiotherapy or treatment with gonadotrophin-releasing hormone analogues. In the absence of surgery, induced menopause may be permanent or temporary.

Stages of reproductive ageing

A staging system that uses the final or last menstrual period (FMP) as the anchor to describe reproductive ageing was proposed by the Stages of Reproductive Aging Workshop. In this system, five stages precede and two stages follow the final menstrual period (Figure 1.2). Stages –5 to –3 encompass the reproductive interval, stages –2 and –1 are the menopausal transition and stages 1 and 2 are the postmenopause. After menarche (entry into stage –5), it usually takes several years for regular menstrual cycles to become established. Menstrual periods should then occur every 21–35 days for a number of years (stages –4 and –3). A woman's menstrual cycles remain regular in stage –2 (early menopausal transition) but the duration changes by seven days or more (cycles are now every 24 days instead of every 31 days). Stage –1 (late menopausal transition) is characterized by two or more missed periods and at least one intermenstrual interval of 60 days or more. Stages +1 (early) and +2 (late) encompass the postmenopause. The early postmenopause is defined as five years since the FMP and the late postmenopause thereafter until death.

Stages:	−5	−4	−3	−2	−1	0	+1	+2
Terminology:	Reproductive			Menopausal transition			Postmenopause	
	Early	Peak	Late	Early	Late*		Early*	Late
				Perimenopause				
Duration of stages:	Variable			Variable			a: 1 year; b: 4 yrs	Until demise
Menstrual cycles:	Variable to regular	Regular		Variable cycle length (>7 days different from normal)	≥2 skipped cycles and an interval of amenorrhoea (≥60 days)	Amen = 12 mos	None	
Endocrine:	normal FSH	↑FSH	↑FSH	↑FSH	↑FSH		↑FSH	

Final menstrual period (FMP) — indicated at stage 0

* Stages most likely to be characterized by vasomotor symptoms   ↑ = elevated

Figure 1.2 STRAW staging system for reproductive ageing. Reprinted from Soules MR *et al.* (2001), with permission from American Society for Reproductive Medicine

Ovarian function

The main steroid hormones produced by the ovary are oestradiol, progesterone and testosterone. In premenopausal women, ovarian function is controlled by the two pituitary gonadotrophins: follicle-stimulating hormone (FSH) and luteinizing hormone (LH). Follicle-stimulating hormone itself is controlled primarily by the pulsatile secretion of hypothalamic gonadotrophin-releasing hormone (GnRH) and is modulated by the negative feedback of oestradiol and progesterone and the ovarian peptide inhibin. Measurement of the levels of FSH to determine the efficacy of hormone

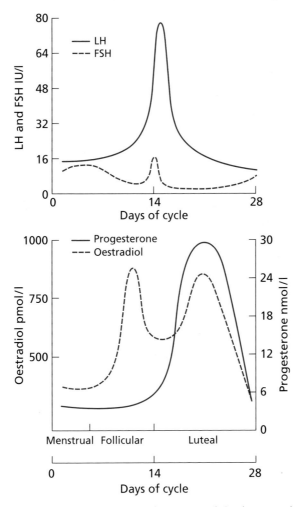

Figure 1.3 Levels of gonadotrophin, oestradiol and progesterone during the menstrual cycle

replacement therapy is thus of little value, as this gonadotrophin is also controlled by the ovarian peptide inhibin (see Chapter 5). Luteinizing hormone is under the principal control of GnRH, with negative feedback control from oestradiol and progesterone for most of the cycle; positive oestradiol feedback generates the mid-cycle surge in levels of LH that in turn triggers ovulation (Figure 1.3).

Each ovary receives a finite endowment of oocytes, the numbers of which are maximal at 20–28 weeks of intrauterine life. From mid-gestation onwards, a logarithmic reduction in these germ cells occurs until, some 50 years later, the stock of oocytes becomes exhausted. The ovary gradually becomes less responsive to gonadotrophins several years before menses cease. This results in a reduction in production of oestrogen and an increase in levels of gonadotrophin. There is thus a gradual increase in circulating levels of FSH and later of LH and a decrease in levels of oestradiol and inhibin. Levels of FSH fluctuate markedly from premenopausal to postmenopausal values on virtually a daily basis during the menopausal transition (Figure 1.4). Their diagnostic use is thus severely limited (see Chapter 5). These changes in circulating levels of hormones frequently occur in the face of ovulatory menstrual cycles. As ovarian unresponsiveness becomes more marked, cycles tend to become anovulatory, and complete failure of follicular development eventually occurs. Production of oestradiol, which occurs in the granulosa and theca cells that surround the oocyte, is no longer sufficient to stimulate the endometrium, and amenorrhoea then ensues, with levels of FSH and LH now persistently elevated. Levels of FSH >30 IU/l are generally considered to be in the postmenopausal range.

The ovaries are an important source of testosterone, which is hydroxylated to dihydrotestosterone. Testosterone can also be aromatized to oestradiol. Precursor oestrogen hormones, such as androstenedione and dehydroepiandrosterone

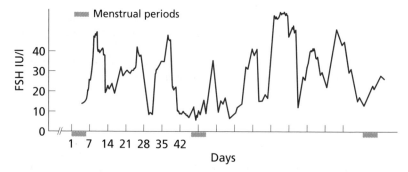

Figure 1.4 Levels of follicle-stimulating hormone during the menopause

(DHEA), are produced in the ovaries and the adrenals, and both possess a less potent androgenic effect than testosterone. By the time women reach their mid-40s, mean circulating levels of testosterone, androstenedione, DHEA and the sulphate product (DHEA-S) are approximately half those of women in their 20s. Menopausal status does not affect levels of androgens in women aged 45–54 years, however, and the postmenopausal ovary seems to be an ongoing site of testosterone production. Low circulating levels of androgens have been proposed to be associated with low sexual desire; however, no level of a single androgen is predictive of low sexual function in women.

Further reading

Demography

Cresswell JL, Egger P, Fall CH, et al. Is the age of menopause determined in utero? Early Hum Dev 1997;**49**:143–8.

Elias SG, van Noord PA, Peeters PH, et al. Caloric restriction reduces age at menopause: the effect of the 1944–1945 Dutch famine. Menopause 2003;**10**: 399–405.

Gold EB, Bromberger J, Crawford S, et al. Factors associated with age at natural menopause in a multiethnic sample of midlife women. Am J Epidemiol 2001; **153**:865–74.

Hardy R, Kuh D. Social and environmental conditions across the life course and age at menopause in a British birth cohort study. BJOG 2005;**112**:346–54.

Lawlor DA, Ebrahim S, Smith GD. The association of socio-economic position across the life course and age at menopause: the British Women's Heart and Health Study. BJOG 2003;**110**:1078–87.

Office for National Statistics and Government Actuaries Department, UK. http://www.gad.gov.uk (last accessed 21 October 2005).

Reynolds RF, Obermeyer CM. Age at natural menopause in Spain and the United States: results from the DAMES project. Am J Hum Biol 2005;**17**:331–40.

Seltzer GB, Schupf N, Wu HS. A prospective study of menopause in women with Down's syndrome. J Intellect Disabil Res 2001;**45**:1–7.

US Census Bureau. Global Population at a Glance: 2002 and Beyond. Washington, DC: US Census Bureau, 2004. Available at: http://www.census.gov/ipc/ (last accessed 29 September 2005).

van Asselt KM, Kok HS, van Der Schouw YT, et al. Current smoking at menopause rather than duration determines the onset of natural menopause. Epidemiology 2004;**15**:634–9.

Endocrinology/ovarian function

Bachmann G, Bancroft J, Braunstein G, et al. Female androgen insufficiency: the Princeton consensus statement on definition, classification, and assessment. Fertil Steril 2002;**77**:660–5.

Davis SR, Davison SK, Donath S, *et al.* Circulating androgen levels and self-reported sexual function in women. *JAMA* 2005;**294**:91–6.

Davison S, Bell R, Donath S, *et al.* Androgen levels in adult females: changes with age, menopause and oophorectomy. *J Clin Endocrinol Metab* 2005;**90**:3847–53.

Guay A, Munarriz R, Jacobson J, *et al.* Serum androgen levels in healthy premenopausal women with and without sexual dysfunction: part A. Serum androgen levels in women aged 20–49 years with no complaints of sexual dysfunction. *Int J Impotence Res* 2004:**16**:112–20.

Landgren BM, Collins A, Csemiczky G, *et al.* Menopause transition: annual changes in serum hormonal patterns over the menstrual cycle in women during a nine-year period prior to menopause. *J Clin Endocrinol Metab* 2004;**89**:2763–9.

Soules MR, Sherman S, Parrott E, *et al.* Executive summary: Stages of Reproductive Aging Workshop (STRAW). *Fertil Steril* 2001;**76**:874–8.

Treloar AE, Boynton RE, Behn BG, Brown BW. Variation of the human menstrual cycle through reproductive life. *Int J Fertil* 1967;**12**:77–126

Utian WH. The international menopause society menopause-related terminology definitions. *Climacteric* 1999;**2**:284–6.

WHO Scientific Group. *Research on Menopause in the 1990s. Report of a WHO Scientific Group. WHO Technical Report Series 866.* Geneva: World Health Organization, 1996.

2 Menopausal symptoms

Vasomotor symptoms
Sexual dysfunction
Psychological symptoms
Further reading

The change in hormone levels that occurs during the climacteric, particularly the decline in levels of oestrogen, can cause acute menopausal symptoms. About 70% of women in Western cultures will experience vasomotor symptoms, such as hot flushes and night sweats. Some women also report psychological symptoms, which can be related to their experience of vasomotor symptoms or menstrual changes or to concurrent life events. These include tiredness, depressed mood, loss of libido, lethargy and arthralgia. Cultural differences in attitudes to the menopause seem to exist: for example, menopausal complaints are fewer in Japanese women than in North American women. Although women with a higher level of education seem to have fewer symptoms, evidence about the effect of exercise is conflicting.

Vasomotor symptoms

Hot flushes and night sweats are the most common symptoms of the menopause, and, although they may begin before periods stop, the prevalence of flushes is highest in the first year after the final menstrual period. Although they are usually present for less than five years, some women will continue to flush beyond the age of 60 years. Flushes are episodes of inappropriate heat loss mediated by cutaneous vasodilation over the upper trunk. Sympathetic nervous control of blood flow in the skin is impaired in women with menopausal flushes, in whom reflex constriction to an ice stimulus cannot be elicited. More recently, serotonin and its receptors in the central nervous system have been implicated.

Hot flushes can occur at any time of the day, and normal sleep patterns may be disturbed at night. Chronically disturbed sleep, in turn, can lead to insomnia, irritability and difficulties with short-term memory and concentration.

Sexual dysfunction

Changes in sexual behaviour and activity are not uncommon in menopausal women, and this is attracting much research attention. Interest in sexual activities declines in both sexes with increasing age, and this change seems to be more pronounced in women. The US National Health and Social Life

Table 2.1

Consensus classification system. Adapted from Basson (2000)

Classification	Definition
I Sexual desire disorders	
A Hypoactive sexual desire disorder (HSDD)	The persistent or recurrent deficiency (or absence) of sexual fantasies/thoughts and/or desire for or receptivity to sexual activity, which causes personal distress
B Sexual aversion disorder (SAD)	The persistent or recurrent phobic aversion and avoidance of sexual contact with a sexual partner, which causes personal distress
II Sexual arousal disorders	The persistent or recurrent inability to attain or maintain sufficient sexual excitement, causing personal distress, which may be expressed as a lack of subjective excitement, or genital (lubrication/swelling) or other somatic responses
III Orgasmic disorder	The persistent or recurrent difficulty, delay in or absence of attaining orgasm after sufficient sexual stimulation and arousal, which causes personal distress
IV Sexual pain disorders	
A Dyspareunia	The recurrent or persistent genital pain associated with sexual intercourse
B Vaginismus	The recurrent or persistent involuntary spasm of the musculature of the outer third of the vagina, which interferes with vaginal penetration and causes personal distress
C Non-coital sexual pain disorders	Recurrent or persistent genital pain induced by non-coital sexual stimulation

Each of the categories above is subtyped on the basis of the medical history, physical examination and laboratory tests as: (A) lifelong versus acquired; (B) generalized versus situational or (C) aetiology (organic, psychogenic, mixed or unknown)

Survey, which was undertaken in people aged 18–59 years, reported that sexual dysfunction is more prevalent for women (43%) than men (31%). Further population studies show that the percentage of women with scores that indicate sexual dysfunction rises from 42% to 88% during the early to late menopausal transition.

The term female sexual dysfunction (FSD) is used now. In 2000, the International Consensus Development Conference on Female Sexual Dysfunction produced a classification system to provide a basis for research of prevalence, aetiology and therapy (Table 2.1).

In reality, these categories often overlap, and one may cause the other. For example, painful intercourse is likely to lead to avoidance of sexual activity, and anticipation of pain leads to lack of arousal, loss of orgasm and an increased chance of pain recurring.

The underlying reasons for FSD are commonly multifactorial. For example, vaginal dryness, which results from declining levels of oestrogen, can cause dyspareunia. Reduced levels of oestrogen can impair peripheral sensory perception, and women may experience discomfort after contact with the skin by clothes or their partner. Non-hormonal factors, such as conflict between partners, insomnia, inadequate stimulation, life stress or depression, however, are important contributors to a woman's level of interest in sexual activity. In addition, male sexual problems – for example, loss of libido and erectile difficulties – should not be overlooked.

Psychological symptoms

Psychological symptoms, including depressed mood, anxiety, irritability, mood swings, lethargy and lack of energy, have been associated with the menopause. General population studies, however, suggest that most women do not experience major changes in mood during the menopausal transition.

Prospective epidemiological studies suggest that psychological problems reported during the menopause are likely to be associated with past problems and current life stresses. It is important, therefore, to take account of other factors, such as prior negative mood, history of premenstrual complaints, negative attitudes toward ageing or the menopause and poor health. In the past, the emphasis was on a woman's change of role – for example, the result of an 'empty nest'. In contrast, a wide range of other issues are relevant to women today (Box 2.1).

These physical and life changes can combine to make a woman feel that she is unable to cope. It is essential that these feelings are recognized and that the woman is offered the opportunity to discuss and clarify their possible causes in her particular case. Treatment, if requested, should be targeted to the individual needs of the woman.

Box 2.1

Factors associated with menopausal psychological symptoms

- Ageing parents and their possible increasing dependency
- Death of a parent, relative or friend
- Loss of partner through death, separation or divorce
- Lack of social support
- Educational or marital difficulties of young adult offspring
- Ill health
- Demanding workload or threat of redundancy
- Economic problems
- Coming to terms with ageing in a culture that values youth and fertility
- Vasomotor instability leading to sleep problems and tiredness

---

Further reading

General symptoms

Aiello EJ, Yasui Y, Tworoger SS, et al. Effect of a yearlong, moderate-intensity exercise intervention on the occurrence and severity of menopause symptoms in postmenopausal women. *Menopause* 2004;11:382–8.

Li C, Samsioe G, Borgfeldt C, et al. Menopause-related symptoms: what are the background factors? A prospective population-based cohort study of Swedish women (The Women's Health in Lund Area study). *Am J Obstet Gynecol* 2003;189:1646–53.

Lock M. Symptom reporting at menopause: a review of cross-cultural findings. *J Br Menopause Soc* 2002;8:132–6.

Vasomotor symptoms

Berendsen HH. The role of serotonin in hot flushes. *Maturitas* 2000;36:155–64.

Rees MCP, Barlow DH. Absence of sustained reflex vasoconstriction in women with menopausal flushes. *Hum Reprod* 1988;3:823–5.

Female sexual dysfunction

Basson R. Women's sexual dysfunctions: revised and expanded. *Sex Relat Therap* 2004;19(Suppl 1):34,S31.

Basson R, Leiblum S, Brotto L, et al. Definitions of women's sexual dysfunction reconsidered: advocating expansion and revision. *J Psychosom Obstet Gynaecol* 2003;24:221–9.

Basson R, Berman J, Burnett A, et al. Report of the international consensus development conference on female sexual dysfunction: definitions and classifications. *J Urol* 2000;163:888–93.

Dennerstein L, Alexander JL, Kotz K. The menopause and sexual functioning: a review of the population-based studies. *Annu Rev Sex Res* 2003;14:64–82.

Laumann EO, Paik A, Rosen RC. Sexual dysfunction in the United States: prevalence and predictors. *JAMA* 1998;**281**:537–44.

Psychological symptoms

Dennerstein L, Guthrie JR, Clark M, *et al*. A population-based study of depressed mood in middle-aged, Australian-born women. *Menopause* 2004;**11**:563–8.

Freeman EW, Sammel MD, Liu L, *et al*. Hormones and menopausal status as predictors of depression in women in transition to menopause. *Arch Gen Psychiatry* 2004;**61**:62–70.

Schmidt PJ, Haq N, Rubinow DR. A longitudinal evaluation of the relationship between reproductive status and mood in perimenopausal women. *Am J Psychiatry* 2004;**161**:2238–44.

3 Chronic conditions affecting postmenopausal health

Osteoporosis
Cardiovascular disease
Dementia
Urogenital atrophy
Further reading

The long-term complications of ageing and oestrogen deficiency may have greater bearing on a woman's quality, and even quantity, of life than the acute short-term symptoms at the time of the menopause. Although they remain clinically silent for many years, they may present a far greater problem in terms of morbidity, mortality and economic burden. Cardiovascular disease is the leading cause of death in women in Western societies (Table 3.1).

Table 3.1

Causes of death in women older than 50 years in England and Wales in 2003. Source: Department of Health (2003)

Condition	ICD-10 code	Age range (years)				
		50–59	60–69	70–79	80–89	≥90
Ischaemic heart disease	I20–I25	1109	3372	10,383	19,757	9315
Cerebrovascular disease	I60–69	725	1614	6588	16,559	9845
Dementia	F01, F03	14	96	1062	4748	3863
Endometrial cancer	C54.1	73	203	288	257	76
Ovarian cancer	C56	634	1019	1141	796	173
Colon cancer	C18	349	658	1310	1558	530
Cancer bronchus and lung	C34	1188	2397	4338	2932	404
Breast cancer	C50	1825	1988	2555	2506	1113
Osteoporosis with pathological fracture	M80	1	17	114	435	446
Pulmonary embolism	I26	86	180	475	889	279
Transport accidents	V01–V99	69	69	106	113	12

Osteoporosis

Osteoporosis affects one in three women and one in 12 men. It is defined in a National Institute of Health consensus statement as 'a skeletal disorder characterized by compromised bone strength predisposing to an increased risk of fracture'. Bone strength reflects the integration of two main features: bone density and bone quality. Bone density is expressed as grams of mineral per area or volume and, in any given individual, is determined by peak bone mass and amount of bone loss. Bone quality refers to architecture, turnover, damage accumulation (for example, microfractures) and mineralization. A fracture occurs when a failure-inducing force, which may or may not involve trauma, is applied to osteoporotic bone. Thus, osteoporosis is a significant risk factor for fracture, and a distinction between risk factors that affect bone metabolism and risk factors for fracture must be made (Figure 3.1). Fractures of the wrist, hip and vertebrae are the main clinical manifestations of osteoporosis, but it is now known that fractures at all skeletal sites (except only the skull and digits) should be regarded as suspicious. Fractures have a major impact on quality of life, result in a significant economic burden and, particularly in the case of hip fractures, are associated with considerable excess mortality. Population demographics predict that the number of osteoporotic fractures will double by 2040.

Bone mineral density

On the basis of the measurement of bone mineral density (BMD) (Table 3.2), the World Health Organization's definitions, applied to post-

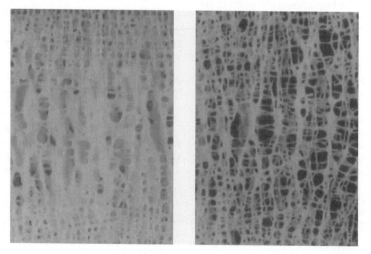

Figure 3.1 Normal (left) and osteoporotic bone (right)

Table 3.2

Definitions of osteoporosis according to the World Health Organization

Description	Definition
Normal	A person has a BMD value between –1 SD and +1 SD of the young adult mean (T score –1 to +1)
Osteopenia	A person has a BMD reduced between –1 and –2.5 SD from the young adult mean (T score –1 to –2.5)
Osteoporosis	A person has a BMD reduced by equal to or more than –2.5 SD from the young adult mean (T score –2.5 or lower)

menopausal women, result in 30% of this population being classified as having osteoporosis. Severe osteoporosis is defined as the presence of a fragility or minimal trauma fracture (fracture after a fall from a chair or standing) and low BMD (T score less than –2.5). The T score is that number of standard deviations (SD) by which the bone in question differs from the young normal mean. Although BMD is a major contributor to risk, other factors, including age, body mass index (BMI), falls, bone quality and rate of bone resorption and formation, play a part in determining whether a person will get a fracture.

Determinants of bone mass

Age
Bone density increases during the growth periods of the teenage years, reaching a peak sometime during the mid-20s. Peak bone density is then sustained for some years and begins to decline during the mid-40s. After the menopause, an accelerated period of bone loss occurs, which lasts for 6–10 years. Thereafter, bone loss continues but at a much slower rate (Figure 3.2). Any bone has a 'threshold' value of bone mass below which the bone will fracture after minor trauma.

Whether a postmenopausal woman develops osteoporosis is determined largely by her peak bone mass, rate of postmenopausal bone loss and longevity. One of the reasons men generally develop osteoporosis only late in life is because they have a much higher peak bone mass than women and do not have the accelerated decade of loss consequent on the female endocrine menopause. Intuitively, some of the measures to prevent osteoporosis would include encouragement in childhood and adolescence of a diet replete in calcium and vitamin D coupled with weight-bearing exercise and discouragement of smoking to enhance peak bone mass. Studies are required, however, to examine the efficacy of these interventions.

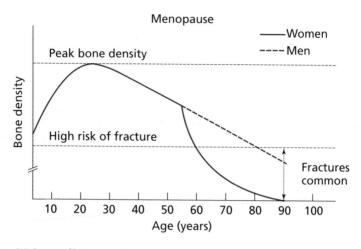

Figure 3.2 Pattern of bone mass with age

Ethnicity and genetic factors

An ethnic variation in the susceptibility to osteoporosis exists, with Caucasian women, for example, having a higher rate of fracture than those of African-Caribbean origin. It is unlikely that a single gene defect exists for osteoporosis, but several candidates that influence BMD have been examined, including those for the vitamin D receptor, oestrogen receptor and collagen. General agreement, however, is that bone density is determined largely by genetic factors, with environmental influences playing a lesser role.

Depot medroxyprogesterone acetate contraception

The relation between BMD and the use of depot medroxyprogesterone acetate (DMPA) is complex. The best available evidence suggests that the amenorrhoea induced by DMPA contraception is associated with a 5–10% loss of bone, which, however, is not progressive. Much depends on the patient's risk factors for osteoporosis. Thus, if, for example, a woman of normal build with a good diet and exercise pattern, she is probably safe, but, conversely, if she has a family history of osteoporosis and a personal history of poor diet and exercise and cigarette consumption, an estimate of bone density should be obtained. If the results are in the osteopenic range, an alternative means of contraception should be considered. In any case, DMPA probably should be discontinued at age 40 years to allow resumption of ovarian cycling for the remaining 10 years or so up to the natural menopause. The long-term skeletal effects of DMPA in teenagers who have yet to achieve peak bone mass presently is uncertain and has to be balanced against the benefits of a very effective form of contraception. Any fall in BMD on starting treatment, however, seems to reverse rapidly on stopping DMPA.

Risk factors for the development of osteoporosis

Specific populations at greatly increased risk of osteoporotic fracture can be identified (Table 3.3). Although these risk factors have been useful at a population level, their use in clinical practice to assess an individual's risk of osteoporosis is difficult, as the increased risk with some factors is small. The factors most important in clinical practice to alert the health professional to the possible risk are parental history of fracture (particularly a family history of hip fracture), early menopause, chronic use of corticosteroids (oral and possibly inhaled), prolonged immobilization and prior fracture.

Table 3.3
Risk factors for osteoporosis

Risk factor	Example
Genetic	• Family history of fracture (particularly a first-degree relative with hip fracture)
Constitutional	• Low body mass index
	• Early menopause (<45 years of age)
Environmental	• Cigarette smoking
	• Alcohol abuse
	• Low calcium intake
	• Sedentary lifestyle
Drugs	• Corticosteroids, >5 mg prednisolone or equivalent daily
Diseases	• Rheumatoid arthritis
	• Neuromuscular disease
	• Chronic liver disease
	• Malabsorption syndromes
	• Hyperparathyroidism
	• Hyperthyroidism
	• Hypogonadism

Clinical consequences of osteoporosis

Fractures are the clinical consequences of osteoporosis. The most common sites of osteoporotic fractures are:

- lower end of radius (wrist or Colles' fracture)
- proximal femur (hip)
- vertebrae.

Colles' fractures frequently occur after a fall onto an outstretched hand. Although such fractures seldom require hospitalization, they are very painful and considerably reduce mobility and function. Other sites include pelvis, ribs, humerus and distal femur.

Hip fracture in young patients is usually the result of road traffic accidents. In older patients, however, hip fractures are caused by falls or may even occur spontaneously. The incidence of hip fracture is about twice as high in women as in men. In many Western countries, the remaining lifetime risk of a hip fracture in Caucasian women at the age of menopause is about 14%. Hip fracture is associated with more deaths, disability and medical costs than all other osteoporotic fractures combined. In the year after a hip fracture, mortality is about 30%. Some 50% of patients who survive hip fractures have permanent disability and fail to regain their previous level of independence.

Vertebral fractures are difficult to quantify, as many patients remain asymptomatic until considerable deformity has occurred. Vertebral fractures often present as non-specific back pain and may be undiagnosed for many years. Indeed, as many as nine of 10 such fractures are estimated never to come under medical attention. Vertebral fractures lead to a loss of height and curvature of the spine, with the typical dorsal kyphosis ('dowager's hump'). Multiple fractures may give rise to loss of height, considerable loss of quality of life and ultimately may impair respiratory function. Even one vertebral fracture is a powerful predictor for future vertebral and other osteoporotic fractures. The prevention of the first fracture and the identification of individuals at risk of this is a central goal of research into osteoporosis.

By the age of 80 years, most women will have sustained one or more fractures of varying severity. The National Health Service's annual expenditure on the acute and aftercare of osteoporosis-related fractures is close to £1.7 billion. This figure does not encompass the economic costs of family members diverting from economic activity to caring.

Cardiovascular disease

The term 'cardiovascular disease' (CVD) is used to describe diseases of the heart and associated blood vessels. Myocardial infarction and stroke are the primary clinical endpoints.

Although CVD is rarely the cause of death in women before the sixth decade, it is the most common cause after the age of 60 years (see Table 3.1). Most of the evidence for an atherogenic effect of the menopause comes from animal models and studies of surgically menopausal women. Oophorectomized women are at 2–3-fold higher risk of coronary heart disease (CHD) than age-matched premenopausal women, although some studies that used women who had undergone hysterectomy with conservation of ovaries as controls have found no difference. However these women may have undergone 'silent' early ovarian failure (Chapter 11).

Coronary heart disease

Coronary heart disease, the most common single cause of death in British women, accounts for almost one-quarter of all deaths in women (see Table 3.1), but it is often erroneously considered to be largely a problem of men. Myocardial infarction involves ischaemic damage to the myocardium after blockage to one or more of the coronary arteries (Box 3.1). This is usually the result of atherosclerotic thickening of the vessel, known as plaque, with the superimposition of a thrombus.

The incidence of CHD increases after the menopause, but when age–sex specific rates are examined, the exponential rise is remarkably constant in both sexes and is not affected by the transition through the menopause (Figure 3.3). The sex ratio does not decrease with age, but it persists after the menopause. As the female portion of the elderly population is larger than the male, the age–sex specific death rate may provide a more useful figure than simply the total number of deaths.

Women tend to be 8–10 years older than men at presentation – a factor that may influence therapeutic decisions and responses to treatment. Furthermore, women tend to have more early complications such as tachycardia after a myocardial infarction; a higher mortality after interventions, such as percutaneous coronary intervention or bypass surgery and a lower likelihood of being free from angina than men. Men, however, are far more likely to have a fatal recurrent event than women, despite comparable numbers of events.

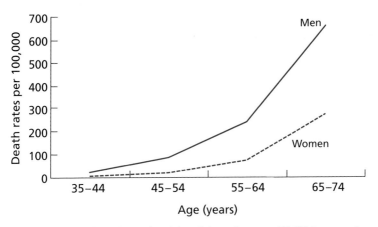

Figure 3.3 Age-sex specific death rates from ischaemic heart disease per 100,000 for men and women in England and Wales. Source: Department of Health (2003)

Box 3.1

Risk factors for myocardial infarction

Lipid profiles
Lipoprotein(a)
Metabolic syndrome
Inflammation
Homocysteine
Smoking
Depression and stress

Risk factors for myocardial infarction

Lipid profiles

Abnormal levels of lipoproteins are a strong risk factor for CVD for men and women, particularly high levels of low-density lipoprotein cholesterol (LDL-C) and combined hyperlipidaemia (increased levels of triglycerides, LDL-C, very-low-density lipoprotein cholesterol [VLDL-C], intermediate-density lipoprotein cholesterol [IDL-C] and small dense LDL-C and low levels of high-density lipoprotein cholesterol [HDL-C]). Because of the decrease in oestrogen production, alterations in lipid metabolism are thought to account for a substantial proportion of the increased risk of CVD seen in postmenopausal women. High levels of total cholesterol and LDL-C are believed to be a stronger risk factor for older women than for men.

Lipoprotein(a)

Although less well known, high serum levels of lipoprotein(a) are becoming recognized as a very important risk factor for CVD. Lipoprotein(a) is a glycoprotein that is associated with apoprotein B; it exaggerates atherogenesis by increasing the deposition of LDL-C in the arterial wall, as well as by inhibiting thrombolysis. In addition, lipoprotein(a) is an antiplasminogen, which accounts for its inhibition of thrombolysis.

Metabolic syndrome

The metabolic syndrome encompasses a range of conditions, including insulin resistance, combined hyperlipidaemia, hypertension, clotting abnormalities, obesity and overt diabetes, that predispose a person to CVD. The features of the metabolic syndrome are more prevalent in women with heart disease than healthy women or men with heart disease. Overt diabetes is associated with a greater increase in risk for atherosclerosis in women than men. This effect may be the result of the relatively more severe dyslipidaemia seen in women with diabetes compared with men with diabetes, particularly in terms of levels of triglycerides. In addition, higher BMI in adulthood is an especially strong risk factor for CHD among women who were small at birth.

Inflammation

Recent advances in our understanding of the role of inflammation in atherogenesis have led to the emergence of new markers for the prediction of coronary events, such as C-reactive protein (CRP), which is an indicator of systemic inflammation. The nested case–control Women's Health Study of 28,263 women showed that CRP was as powerful an independent predictor as any other single factor. Women in the highest quartile of CRP levels had a 5–7-fold increased risk of cardiac and vascular events over a three-year follow-up period.

Homocysteine

Increased plasma levels of total homocysteine have been shown to be an independent risk factor for peripheral and coronary atherosclerosis. People with homocystinuria are at increased risk for vascular disease, and, conversely, patients with atherosclerosis frequently have increased plasma levels of total homocysteine. The underlying mechanisms are uncertain. Increased levels of total homocysteine have been suggested to have a direct effect on the endothelium or to increase vascular uptake of LDL-C.

Smoking

This remains one of the major causal factors for myocardial infarction, and the excess risk of myocardial infarction among smokers is of the order of 400 additional infarctions per million treatment years.

Depression and stress

Acute and chronic stress are thought to trigger myocardial infarction in both sexes by contributing to plaque rupture. Depression seems to be an independent risk factor for poor outcome after acute cardiac events or surgery in women.

Stroke

The incidence of stroke increases with age, doubling in each decade of life after the sixth decade, and stroke is a leading cause of death in women (Box 3.2). One in five 50-year-old Caucasian women in the Western world will develop stroke during their lifetime. Many survivors are left with significant physical and mental impairment and have serious long-term disability. Analogous to the processes involved in myocardial infarction, the most

> **Box 3.2**
>
> Risk factors for stroke
> ___
>
> Hypertension
> Smoking
> Diabetes
> Asymptomatic carotid stenosis
> Atrial fibrillation

common form of stroke involves brain infarction that results from obstruction of the cerebral arteries. Other forms of stroke involve the rupture of aneurysms, which leads to primary intracerebral and subarachnoid haemorrhage.

Risk factors for stroke

Hypertension
This is a major risk factor for both cerebral infarction and intracerebral haemorrhage. The incidence of stroke increases in proportion to systolic and diastolic blood pressures. This relation is 'direct, continuous and apparently independent'. Isolated systolic hypertension (systolic blood pressure >160 mmHg and diastolic blood pressure <90 mmHg) is an important risk factor for stroke in elderly people.

Smoking
Cigarette smoking has long been recognized as a major risk factor for stroke. The relative risk of cerebral infarction in smokers is about double that in non-smokers.

Diabetes
Patients with diabetes have an increased relative risk of stroke, ranging from 1.8- to nearly six-fold. From 1976 to 1980 in the US, a history of stroke was 2.5–4 times more common in people with diabetes than in people with normal glucose tolerance.

Asymptomatic carotid stenosis
About 7–10% of men and 5–7% of women older than 65 years have carotid stenoses >50%.

Atrial fibrillation
This is a common arrhythmia and an important risk factor for stroke, with established effective treatment for stroke prevention. The annual risk of

stroke in unselected patients with non-valvular atrial fibrillation is 3–5%, with the condition responsible for 50% of thromboembolic strokes.

Hyperlipidaemia
Abnormalities in levels of serum lipids have traditionally been regarded as a risk factor for coronary artery disease but not cerebrovascular disease. The relation between lipids and stroke is complex, however, and the risk of stroke and amount of carotid atheroma can be reduced with cholesterol-lowering drugs. A large meta-analysis of 45 prospective observational cohorts involving 450,000 participants found no association between levels of cholesterol and the rate of stroke. These epidemiological studies are confounded by reports of an inverse association between total cholesterol and cerebral haemorrhage, however, with a higher mortality from haemorrhagic stroke among people with low serum levels of cholesterol. Although statins are beneficial in stroke prevention in patients with CHD, their mechanisms of action are uncertain. Although some of the reduction in the rate of stroke may be the result of alterations in lipid levels, statins may also act through mechanisms unrelated to their lipid-lowering properties, such as improved endothelial function; plaque stabilization; and antithrombotic, anti-inflammatory and neuroprotective properties.

Obesity
This predisposes to CVD in general and to stroke in particular. In women, obesity is associated with an increased risk of ischaemic stroke, with rates of stroke increasing with increasing BMI.

Dementia

Dementia is a clinical term used to describe a condition in which a patient has impairment of cognitive faculties, including loss of memory, language, thinking and judgement, which causes significant difficulties in functioning. Its prevalence and incidence increase with age, and the risk of developing dementia doubles every five years after the age of 65 years. About 7% of people older than 65 years are affected; this increases to at least 20% in people older than 80 years and may exceed 50% in people older than 90 years.

In the UK, an estimated 750,000 people have dementia; this includes more than 18,000 people younger than 65 years. Four to five million people in the US and 25 million worldwide have dementia. The prevalence and incidence of dementia show little geographical variation, but, worldwide, most patients with dementia live in less developed regions. As more people are living longer, the total number of people affected will continue to increase, with an estimated 1.8 million affected in the UK by 2050 and 114 million worldwide.

The three common types of dementia are Alzheimer's disease, vascular dementia and dementia with Lewy bodies. The average life expectancy of a person with dementia is 3–7 years after diagnosis, although diagnosis often occurs some years after first onset of symptoms. The World Health Organization recognizes dementia as one of the major causes of disability worldwide. It causes significant distress to patients, their carers and families and has an enormous impact on society. It is important to stress that although cognitive impairment is a central feature of dementia, psychological and behavioural changes are also common and important symptoms. These frequently cause carers stress and are major factors that lead to hospital admission or institutional care, or both. Women have a central role in providing care and support to people with dementia – as a member of a family or as a voluntary or aid carer.

Urogenital atrophy

The lower urinary and genital tracts have a common embryological origin and are approximated closely in adult women. Oestrogen receptors and progesterone receptors are present in the vagina, urethra, bladder and pelvic floor musculature. Oestrogen deficiency after menopause causes atrophic changes within the urogenital tract and is associated with urinary symptoms, such as frequency, urgency, nocturia, incontinence and recurrent infection. These symptoms may co-exist with those of vaginal atrophy, including dyspareunia, itching, burning and dryness (Table 3.4)

Table 3.4
Symptoms of urogenital atrophy

Site of atrophy	Symptoms
Vaginal	• Vaginal dryness • Vaginal burning • Pruritus • Dyspareunia • Prolapse
Urinary	• Urgency • Frequency • Dysuria • Urinary tract infection • Incontinence • Voiding difficulties

Further reading

General

Department of Health. *Series DH2. No. 30. Mortality Statistics Cause Review of the Registrar General on Deaths by Cause, Sex and Age, in England and Wales, 2003.* http://www.statistics.gov.uk (last accessed 4 October 2005).

British Heart Foundation Statistics Website. http://www.heartstats.org (last accessed 14 October 2005).

Osteoporosis

Cauley JA, Lui LY, Stone KL, *et al.* Longitudinal study of changes in hip bone mineral density in Caucasian and African-American women. *J Am Geriatr Soc* 2005; **53**:183–9.

Department of Health. *National Service Framework for Older People.* Wetherby: Department of Health, 2001. Available at: http://www.dh.gov.uk/ (last accessed 5 October 2005).

Israel E, Banerjee TR, Fitzmaurice GM, *et al.* Effects of inhaled glucocorticoids on bone density in premenopausal women. *N Engl J Med* 2001;**345**:941–7.

Kanis JA, Johansson H, Oden A, *et al.* A family history of fracture and fracture risk: a meta-analysis. *Bone* 2004;**35**:1029–37.

Kanis JA, Johansson H, Oden A, *et al.* A meta-analysis of prior corticosteroid use and fracture risk. *J Bone Miner Res* 2004;**19**:893–9.

Kanis JA, Johnell O, De Laet C, *et al.* A meta-analysis of previous fracture and subsequent fracture risk. *Bone* 2004;**35**:375–82.

Langhammer A, Norjavaara E, de Verdier MG, *et al.* Use of inhaled corticosteroids and bone mineral density in a population based study: the Nord-Trondelag Health Study (the HUNT Study). *Pharmacoepidemiol Drug Saf* 2004;**13**:569–79.

Lindsay R, Silverman SL, Cooper C, *et al.* Risk of new vertebral fracture in the year following a fracture. *JAMA* 2001;**285**:320–3.

NIH Consensus Development Panel on Osteoporosis Prevention, Diagnosis, and Therapy. Osteoporosis prevention, diagnosis, and therapy. *JAMA* 2001;**285**:785–95.

Orr-Walker BJ, Evans MC, Ames RW, *et al.* The effect of past use of the injectable contraceptive depot medroxyprogesterone acetate on bone mineral density in normal post-menopausal women. *Clin Endocrinol (Oxf)* 1998;**49**:615–18.

Roberts SE, Goldacre MJ. Time trends and demography of mortality after fractured neck of femur in an English population, 1968–98: database study. *BMJ* 2003;**327**:771–5.

Royal College of Physicians. *Osteoporosis: Clinical Guidelines for Prevention and Treatment.* London: Royal College of Physicians, 1999. http://www.rcplondon.ac.uk (last accessed 5 October 2005).

Royal College of Physicians. *Osteoporosis: Clinical Guidelines for Prevention and Treatment. Update on Pharmacological Interventions and an Algorithm for Management.* London: Royal College of Physicians, 2000. http://www.rcplondon.ac.uk (last accessed 5 October 2005).

Scholes D, LaCroix AZ, Ichikawa LE, *et al.* Change in bone mineral density among adolescent women using and discontinuing depot medroxyprogesterone acetate contraception. *Arch Pediatr Adolesc Med* 2005;**159**:139–44.

van Balen R, Steyerberg EW, Polder JJ, *et al.* Hip fracture in elderly patients: outcomes for function, quality of life, and type of residence. *Clin Orthop* 2001;**390**:232–43.

World Health Organization. *Assessment of Fracture Risk and its Application to Screening for Postmenopausal Osteoporosis. WHO Technical Report Series 843.* Geneva: WHO, 1994.

Cardiovascular disease

Fine-Edelstein JS, Wolf PA, O'Leary DH, *et al.* Precursors of extracranial carotid atherosclerosis in the Framingham Study. *Neurology* 1994;**44**:1046–50.

Goldstein LBM, Adams RM, Becker KM, *et al.* Primary prevention of ischemic stroke: a statement for healthcare professionals from the Stroke Council of the American Heart Association. *Circulation* 2001;**103**:163–82.

Knopp RH. Risk factors for coronary artery disease in women. *Am J Cardiol* 2002;**89**:28E–34E.

Malenka DJ, O'Rourke D, Miller MA, *et al.* Cause of in-hospital death in 12,232 consecutive patients undergoing percutaneous transluminal coronary angioplasty. *Am Heart J* 1999;**137**:632–8.

Qizilbash N, Lewington S, Duffy S, *et al.* Cholesterol, diastolic blood pressure, and stroke: 13,000 strokes in 450,000 people in 45 prospective cohorts: Prospective Studies Collaboration. *Lancet* 1995;**346**:1647–53.

Rich-Edwards JW, Kleinman K, Michels KB, *et al.* Longitudinal study of birth weight and adult body mass index in predicting risk of coronary heart disease and stroke in women. *BMJ* 2005;**330**:1115.

Ridker PM, Hennekens CH, Buring JE, Rifai NC. C-reactive protein and other markers of inflammation in the prediction of cardiovascular disease in women. *N Engl J Med* 2000;**342**:836–43.

Schreiner PJ, Niemela M, Miettinen H, *et al.* Gender differences in recurrent coronary events. The FINMONICA MI register. *Eur Heart J* 2001;**22**:762–8.

Simpson CR, Hannaford PC, Williams D. Evidence for inequalities in the management of coronary heart disease in Scotland. *Heart* 2005;**91**:630–4.

Tunstall-Pedoe H, Morrison C, Woodward M, *et al.* Sex differences in myocardial infarction and coronary deaths in the Scottish MONICA population of Glasgow 1985–1991: presentation, diagnosis, treatment, and 28 day care fatality of 3991 events in men and 1551 events in women. *Circulation* 1996;**93**:1981–92.

Dementia

Langa KM, Foster NL, Larson EB. Mixed dementia: emerging concepts and therapeutic implications. *JAMA* 2004;**292**:2901–8.

Rosenblatt A, Samus QM, Steele CD, *et al.* The Maryland Assisted Living Study: prevalence, recognition, and treatment of dementia and other psychiatric disorders in the assisted living population of central Maryland. *J Am Geriatr Soc* 2004;**52**:1618–25.

Wimo A, Winblad B, Aguero-Torres H, von Strauss E. The magnitude of dementia occurrence in the world. *Alzheimer Dis Assoc Disord* 2003;17:63–7.

Urogenital ageing

Davila GW, Singh A, Karapanagiotou I, *et al.* Are women with urogenital atrophy symptomatic? *Am J Obstet Gynecol* 2003;188:382–8.

Milsom I, Molander U. Urogenital ageing. *J Br Menopause Soc* 1998;4:151–6.

Robinson D, Cardozo LD. The role of estrogens in female lower urinary tract dysfunction. *Urology* 2003;62:45–51.

van Geelen JM, van de Weijer PH, Arnolds HT. Urogenital symptoms and resulting discomfort in non-institutionalized Dutch women aged 50–75 years. *Int Urogynecol J Pelvic Floor Dysfunct* 2000;11:9–14.

Versi E, Harvey MA, Cardozo L, *et al.* Urogenital prolapse and atrophy at menopause: a prevalence study. *Int Urogynecol J Pelvic Floor Dysfunct* 2001;12:107–10.

ASSESSMENT AND INVESTIGATIONS

4 Assessment, contraception and sexual health

Assessment
Examination
Follow up
Contraception
Sexual health
Further reading

Consultations about the menopause are becoming more complex because of the various oestrogen and non-oestrogen-based treatments available and the major controversies that surround hormone replacement therapy (HRT). This chapter describes assessment, follow up, contraception and sexual health.

Assessment

The following details useful information that can be obtained from the patient and underpins any further assessment. It is important to ascertain menopausal status, risk factors for cardiovascular disease and osteoporosis, as well as the woman's personal views on the menopause itself and on any interventions (Box 4.1).

It is a woman's evidence-based patient choice to take or not to take HRT or any therapy, and her decision must be recorded in the notes.

Examination

Physical examination should include recording of body mass index and blood pressure. In March 2001, the UK Committee on Safety of Medicines (CSM) advised that clinical examination of the breasts and pelvic examination are not *routinely* necessary in all women who take HRT, but they must be performed if clinically indicated. These recommendations are in line with those in operation for women who take the oral contraceptive pill.

Women should also be encouraged to participate in the national cervical screening programme, which, in the UK, invites women aged 25–64 years for screening. The national mammography screening programme and personal

Box 4.1

Patient history

Periods, symptoms and contraception
- Date of last menstrual period (could she be pregnant?)
- Frequency, heaviness and duration of periods
- Hot flushes and night sweats
- Vaginal dryness
- Other symptoms
- Contraception

Personal or family medical problems
1. Breast, ovarian or bowel cancer in close family members
   - Have any parents, sisters or brothers or the patient had such cancers?
   - If so, at what age did they develop it?
2. Deep vein thrombosis or pulmonary embolism
   - Have any parents, brothers or sisters or the patient had such conditions?
   - If so, when and why did this happen?
     - Was it after a hip or knee replacement?
     - Was the person on the 'pill' or pregnant?
   - Did they have any test to confirm the clot?
   - Was the clinical suspicion confirmed?
   - Were they treated with anticoagulants such as heparin or warfarin?
3. Risk factors for heart disease and strokes
   - Has the patient already had a heart attack or stroke?
   - Have her parents, brothers or sisters had a myocardial infarction or stroke, and, if so, at what age?
   - Does the patient smoke, and, if so, how many cigarettes a day?
   - Does the patient have hypertension or diabetes?
   - Does the patient have high cholesterol levels?
4. Risk factors for osteoporosis
   - Was the menopause before the age of 45 years?
   - Has the patient taken systemic corticosteroids for six months or longer?
   - Has the patient had anorexia or significant weight loss?
   - Does the patient have a family history of osteoporosis (especially in her mother, grandmother or sister)?
   - Has the patient had low calcium or vitamin D intake or deficiency, or malabsorption disorders?
   - Has the patient already had a fracture? If so, was it from standing height, how did it happen and where was it?
5. Other
   - Has the patient had migraines?
   - What medicines are being taken, including herbal remedies and vitamin supplements?
   - Is the patient at risk of pregnancy?
6. What does the patient want?
   - Does she want to take HRT?
   - If yes, what preparation would she prefer - and by what route?
   - If not, what are her most important treatment endpoints?

breast awareness must be discussed. In the UK, the national mammography screening programme invites all women age 50–64 for mammography every three years. Furthermore, the UK National Health Service Cancer Plan recommends that mammographic screening be extended to all women aged 65–70 years and be available on request to women older than 70 years.

The words 'clinically indicated' for pelvic examination should relate to past or current disease, symptoms or family history. It is important not to miss a breast or a pelvic mass, or a pregnancy.

Follow up

After instigating a particular type of treatment, the patient should be seen for follow up after about three months. This is because most symptoms will have responded to oestrogen or non-oestrogen-based treatments by this time. In addition, persistence of any side-effects will be apparent. At three months, the practitioner can decide on the management of residual difficulties. Controversy surrounds the frequency of follow up thereafter. In the UK, the Committee on Safety of Medicines recommends that HRT 'should be re-evaluated at least annually in light of new knowledge and any changes in a woman's risk factors'. It is probably prudent to arrange annual follow up for any treatment (both oestrogen and non-oestrogen-based), as the risks and benefits of any particular strategy for each individual woman will alter with time and need to be discussed. The need for oestrogen often declines with age.

Monitoring of blood pressure is not needed routinely in women who use HRT. Studies of the effects of natural oestrogens have found slight increases and decreases in blood pressure. In general, blood pressure does not change. On rare occasions, conjugated equine oestrogens cause severe hypertension, but this returns to normal when treatment is stopped. In patients whose pre-existing hypertension has been treated to normalize or reduce blood pressure, oestrogens can be given safely (see Chapter 12). Blood pressure should be monitored regularly at six-monthly intervals, as would be good clinical practice in any patient with hypertension. Postmenopausal bleeding and any abnormal bleeding, whether women are taking HRT or not, should always be taken seriously and are indications for specialist referral. It is essential to investigate for cervical or uterine cancer.

Contraception

Perimenopausal women cannot be assumed to be infertile, and there are well documented records of births to women in their 50s. The oldest woman known to have given birth after a spontaneous conception was aged 57 years and 129 days. When an unplanned pregnancy occurs, it can be a disaster: both abortion and childbirth are associated with a higher morbidity and mortality in this age group. Older women have a higher risk of hypertension induced by pregnancy and gestational diabetes. The risk of fetal malformation increases, with an increase in chromosomal disorders such as Down's syndrome, as does the risk of miscarriage. Contraceptive options thus must be considered carefully.

Duration of contraceptive use in the perimenopause

The normal recommendation is to continue contraception after the final menstrual period for at least two years if the woman is younger than 50 years and at least one year if she is older than 50 years old. The final menstrual period can be identified only retrospectively and may be difficult to identify in women who use a contraceptive method that renders them amenorrhoeic and in those who take a combined oral contraceptive or monthly sequential HRT, which induce a cyclical withdrawal bleed. Elevated levels of follicle-stimulating hormone (FSH) after stopping oral contraceptives or HRT do not reliably indicate infertility. Hormone replacement therapy does not provide contraception.

Contraceptive options in the perimenopause

A variety of contraceptive methods are available and their suitability for perimenopausal women is detailed below.

Natural family planning
- This is not appropriate during the menopausal transition.
- It can produce unpredictable cycles, inconsistent temperature changes and atypical mucous changes.
- Methods that rely on the detection of the hormonal changes at ovulation are unreliable.

Coitus interruptus
- This is unreliable but is a method of choice for some couples.
- Vaginal dryness, fear of pregnancy and concomitant changes in libido and potency may alter acceptability.

Condoms
- Ongoing use is acceptable but may cause discomfort.
- The risk of rupture is increased in association with mucosal atrophic changes.
- Lubricating or spermicidal gels should be recommended.

Diaphragm
- Continuation of use is acceptable.

- Mucosal atrophy or prolapse of the vaginal wall, or both, may cause difficulties with fitting or retention.

Note: Some vaginal preparations, including oestrogen creams and pessaries, may damage the rubber used in condoms and diaphragms, which can lead to an increased risk of rupture.

Spermicides
- These may help lubrication, and their efficacy increases with age.
- They should be used with barrier methods or as a single method, eg foams.
- Vaginal atrophic changes can lead to increased sensitivity with mucosal inflammation and breakdown.

Intrauterine devices
- Ongoing use is appropriate if already *in situ* at the time of the menopause, and they may be left in for more than five years until contraception is no longer required.
- They may increase the incidence of abnormal bleeding.

Intrauterine systems
- Intrauterine devices that contain progestogen suppress the endometrium, which leads to amenorrhoea in many women and can be used to treat menorrhagia.
- They may be used in conjunction with oestrogen and could provide 'period free' HRT in the perimenopause.

Combined contraception (oral, patch and vaginal ring)
- Low-dose, combined contraceptives that contain synthetic oestrogens provide reliable contraception, as well as benefits of oestrogen replacement in older women.
- Women who do not smoke, are normotensive, are not overweight and have a benign family history can continue low-dose combined pills until at least their mid-40s or early 50s.
- Synthetic oestrogens may potentiate the age-related increase in cardiovascular and cerebrovascular disease.
- The risk of breast cancer may be slightly increased.

Progestogen-only pills
- These are suitable for use throughout the perimenopause, with no upper age limit for their use.
- Their efficacy improves with age.
- Their use in combination with HRT has not been well evaluated.

Intramuscular progestogens and subdermal progestogens
• Amenorrhoea makes it difficult to identify the menopause.
• Other details are as for progestogen-only pills.

Sterilization (male or female)
• This is the most common form of pregnancy prevention in perimenopausal women in some countries such as the UK.

Sexual health

Traditionally, postmenopausal women are not perceived to be at risk of sexually transmitted infections (STIs). This is because older women are perceived to be relatively sexually inactive and assumed to be in a monogamous heterosexual relationship. As increasing numbers of relationships break down and partners change, such women are at potential risk of acquiring STIs. As postmenopausal women no longer need contraception, the use of barrier methods is infrequent, which further increases their risk.

Scale of the problem

In the US, data from the Centers for Disease Control and Prevention (CDC) show a consistently increasing number of older adults who are being infected with STIs, particularly HIV/AIDS. The cumulative number of cases of HIV/AIDS thus reported to the CDC in adults aged 50 years or older quintupled from 16,288 in 1990 to 90,513 by the end of December 2001. The most rapidly growing group of patients with HIV/AIDS are those who acquire infection through heterosexual contact.

Within the UK, data are available for women who attend genitourinary medicine (GUM) clinics; in 2003, 2601 women aged ≥45 years were diagnosed with a range of STIs (Table 4.1). These figures do not include older women managed for STIs outside of GUM clinics or women with other conditions, for whom a breakdown of diagnoses by age is not available. In the years between 1995 and 2003, some of these infections have shown marked increases in women aged 45 to 64 years, with infectious syphilis increasing by 275%, chlamydial infections by 175% and gonorrhoea by 254%.

Presentation

Postmenopausal women present with a variety of symptoms that may be attributed to oestrogen deficiency or an STI. Often a delay in symptom recognition and healthcare presentation occurs. Older adults are thus more likely to present with advanced HIV disease, including AIDS, compared with

Table 4.1

Selected STIs seen in GUM clinics in 2003 in England, Wales and Northern Ireland, by age. Source: Health Protection Agency (2004)

Condition	Sex	Age group (years)		
		35–44	45–64	>64
Primary and secondary infectious syphilis	Male	474	227	14
	Female	27	15	1
Uncomplicated gonorrhoea	Male	2986	1082	53
	Female	548	138	2
Uncomplicated chlamydial infection	Male	4017	996	57
	Female	2052	412	24
Anogenital herpes simplex (first attack)	Male	1519	624	51
	Female	1518	739	18
Anogenital warts (first attack)	Male	5116	2075	151
	Female	2809	1196	56

their younger counterparts (36% versus 5%). In older adults, suspicion of HIV is often lacking among patients and doctors, and the pre-AIDS phase is shorter and less symptomatic. Clinical deterioration is more rapid among elderly people infected with HIV than among younger adults. The effect of the menopause and older age on HIV disease progression is still unclear, but it may be related to the decreased immune function that accompanies advancing age.

Role of the nurse

Nurses can have an effective impact in a number of ways in both primary and secondary care.

Provision of information

Information resources include books, leaflets and the internet. Nurses can help assess which are best for each woman. The key to good management is individual counselling, which can reinforce basic information, make it relevant to that woman and provide realistic expectations of treatment. It builds a rapport between nurse and patient.

Care and monitoring of menopausal women

Nurses cover the same parameters as doctors but with a different emphasis. Women could see practice nurses at alternate visits. Nurses can provide an informal telephone helpline.

Promoting health in the postmenopausal population
In primary care, nurses can help promote an early foundation of good dietary and lifestyle habits in the young. They may then highlight aspects that need modifying in menopausal women.

Identifying risk factors
Nurses can identify systematically women at increased risk of coronary heart disease or osteoporosis for treatment. A record of the date of the last menstrual period when cervical smears are taken can be used to assess premature ovarian failure. The screening programme can also be used to identify young hysterectomized women who are at risk of early ovarian failure (see Chapter 11). The use of steroids, and the presence of diabetes and hypertension can be identified using computerized records.

Further reading

Contraception

Faculty of Family Planning and Reproductive Health Care Clinical Effectiveness Unit. Contraception for women aged over 40 years. *J Fam Plann Reprod Health Care* 2005;**31**:51–64.

Gebbie A. Contraception in the perimenopause. In: Tomlinson JM, Rees M, Mander A, eds. *Sexual Health and the Menopause*. London: RSM Press, 2005:47–54.

Practice Committee, American Society for Reproductive Medicine. Hormonal contraception: recent advances and controversies. *Fertil Steril* 2004;**82**:520–6.

Sexual health

Centers for Disease Control and Prevention. *AIDS Public Use Data Set through Year-End 2000*. Atlanta: Centers for Disease Control and Prevention, 2000. Database available at: http://www.cdc.gov/ (last accessed 4 October 2005).

Gott CM. Sexual activity and risk-taking in later life. *Health Soc Care Community* 2001;**9**:72–8.

Gott CM, Rogstad KE, Riley V, Ahmed-Jushuf I. Delay in symptom presentation among a sample of older GUM clinic attendees. *Int J STD AIDS* 1999;**10**:43–6.

Health Protection Agency. *Diagnoses of Selected STIs, by Region, Age and Sex seen at GUM Clinics. National Level Summary Tables, 1995–2003*. London: Health Protection Agency, 2004. Available at: www.hpa.org.uk (last accessed 4 October 2005)

Mack KA, Ory MG. AIDS and older Americans at the end of the twentieth century. *J Acquir Immune Defic Syndr* 2003;**33**:68–75.

Mahar F, Sherrard J. Sexually transmitted infections. In: Tomlinson JM, Rees M, Mander A, eds. *Sexual Health and the Menopause*. London: RSM Press, 2005:55–62.

5 Investigations

Endocrine investigations

Levels of follicle-stimulating hormone (FSH) are helpful only if the diagnosis of climacteric symptoms is in doubt and the levels are reported in the menopausal range (>30 IU/l). In the perimenopause, the daily variation in levels of FSH renders this parameter of limited value (see Chapter 1). Levels of FSH do not predict when the last menstrual period will occur and are not a guide to fertility status, as increased levels can occur in the presence of ovulatory cycles. Levels of FSH are of little value in monitoring hormone replacement therapy (HRT), as this gonadotrophin is controlled by inhibin as well as oestradiol in normal physiology. It does need to be measured, however, in women with suspected premature ovarian failure, whether or not they are hysterectomized. The blood sample is best collected on days 3–5 of the cycle (day 1 is the first day of menstruation). Where this is not possible – such as in women with oligomenorrhoea or amenorrhoea or women who have undergone hysterectomy – two samples separated by an interval of two weeks should be obtained.

Estimates of the levels of luteinizing hormone, oestradiol, progesterone and testosterone are of no value in the diagnosis of ovarian failure. Levels of oestradiol may be of some value in checking absorption of oestradiol delivered by the non-oral route. They should not be used, however, when oestrogen is given orally, as the major circulating metabolite in this case is oestrone.

Thyroid function tests (free T4 and thyroid-stimulating hormone)

Abnormalities of thyroid function (which lead to lethargy, weight gain, hair loss and flushes) can often be confused with menopausal symptoms, and thyroid function tests should be done whenever the signs and symptoms are appropriate, particularly if the patient has an inadequate symptomatic response to HRT.

Levels of catecholamines in the urine over 24 hours are used in the diagnosis of phaeochromocytoma – a rare cause of hot flushes. Levels of 5-hydroxyindolacetic acid in urine over 24 hours are used in the diagnosis of carcinoid syndrome – another rare cause of hot flushes. Levels of methylhistamine and red cell tryptase in blood, and of methylhistamine in urine over 24 hours are measured when mastocytosis is suspected; this is a very rare cause of hot flushes.

Testosterone levels

Women who complain of lack of libido may request measurement of levels of testosterone. In women, however, slightly more than two-thirds of circulating testosterone is bound to steroid hormone binding globulin (SHBG) and a further third is weakly bound to albumin, which leaves around 2% of the total testosterone in the free or unbound state. As concentrations of SHBG can fluctuate, total levels of testosterone do not yield meaningful information about exposure of the tissues to androgens. A free testosterone index accurately evaluates the tissue androgen status but is not available routinely in clinical practice.

Risk factors for arterial disease

Factors suitable for assessment in primary care

Simple lipid profiles, for example of total cholesterol, HDL-C, LDL-C and triglycerides, may be useful but only in women with symptoms of arterial disease or a high load of other risk markers.

Factors appropriate for assessment in a specialist clinic or research institute

Detailed lipoprotein profile, including, for example, apolipoproteins AI and B, lipoprotein(a), postprandial lipaemia and lipid peroxidation may be helpful; as may a profile of coagulation and fibrinolysis (such as fibrinogen, factor VII and plasminogen activator inhibitor 1 (PAI-1)), insulin resistance and levels of homocysteine.

Mammography and genetic testing

Mammography

No evidence supports routine mammographic examination of the breasts in women about to start HRT, and no evidence suggests that women on HRT require mammography more frequently than the three-yearly interval offered by the National Health Service Breast Screening Programme (NHSBSP). Observational evidence has shown that exposure to HRT is associated with an increase in breast density on mammography. Randomized placebo-controlled data (including data from the Women's Health Initiative (WHI) and Progestin Estrogen–Progestin Intervention (PEPI) studies), however, have shown that not all HRT regimens have this effect. Unopposed oestrogen (that is, conjugated equine oestrogen) does not seem to induce any increase in density, whereas combined therapy (both cyclical and continuous combined) does, on average, in one in four women who take it. These controlled data have also confirmed that if any increase in density occurs, it all takes place within the first year of exposure, and no evidence shows that duration of use influences this effect. The PEPI and WHI trials additionally reported that the individual degree of increase in density associated with exposure to combined HRT is in the order of 3–6%. Currently, published data from placebo-controlled randomized trials that evaluated the effect of unopposed oestradiol on mammographic density and observational studies are inconsistent. At present, studies suggest that breast density on mammography is unlikely to be affected by current use of HRT in most women who participate in the NHSBSP.

Withdrawal of HRT before mammography has been reported to result in regression of increases in density associated with HRT sufficient to enable more accurate film reading. This question has not been subject to controlled evaluation, but available observational data suggest that this regression of density can occur in as little as two weeks. Interestingly, in the combined HRT component of the WHI study, where women who used HRT were advised to stop their therapy for three months before randomization, no difference was seen in the proportion of abnormal mammograms at baseline, which supports a screening benefit for withdrawal of HRT. The Million Women Study (MWS) contrasts with placebo-controlled evidence as it reported that both unopposed and combined HRT increase density. The MWS investigators additionally concluded, in contrast to all other published evidence, that withdrawal of HRT before screening is unlikely to improve the accuracy of mammography.

By increasing breast density, combined HRT can reduce the sensitivity and specificity of mammography. This would be expected to result in an increase in interval cancers (that is, cancers missed during screening because of decreased sensitivity) and has been reported in observational studies such as the MWS. Interval cancers diagnosed in women who take HRT have not been reported to have more adverse prognostic features, but, again, these data are from uncontrolled studies. Unfortunately, the WHI study, which could help to clarify this question, has not yet provided any information about interval cancers and their biological characteristics. In the combined HRT component of the WHI study, breast cancers associated with HRT were, on average, 2 mm larger and more likely to be lymph-node positive (although this was of borderline significance) than cancers associated with placebo. Predictions of survival on the basis of tumour prognostic variables (that is, size, lymph node involvement and grade) suggest a difference in survival from breast cancer at 10 years of 1.5% in favour of placebo. No information has been published yet about tumour characteristics in the oestrogen-only component of the WHI study.

Genetic testing

The lifetime risk (to 85 years of age) of developing breast cancer in developed countries worldwide is 11% (one in nine). Twenty-seven percent of women are estimated to possibly have an inherited predisposition to breast cancer, but only 3–5% are likely to carry gene faults that confer a substantially increased risk (that is, >50%). Most breast cancers arise in women without a family history and are termed sporadic. In women with a family history (6–19%), this familial association can be the result of chance, environmental factors or genetic predisposition. An inherited risk is likely if the woman has a family member with a young age of onset, has a family with a cluster of cases and a history of bilateral disease in the family. Inherited mutations that affect the BRCA1, BRCA2 and TP53 genes have been identified and have an associated lifetime risk of breast cancer of 80%. Mutations in the BRCA1 and BRCA2 genes account for about one-third of inherited breast cancers. Patients with breast cancer from families who carry mutations have a high risk of cancer in the other breast (>50% by the age of 70 years). The risk of subsequent ovarian cancer is also increased: 44% for women with BRCA1 and 16% for women with BRCA2 by the age of 70 years. A very small proportion (<1%) of breast cancers are associated with rarer cancer predisposition syndromes and germline mutations in genes such as TP53 in Li-Fraumeni syndrome or PTEN in Cowden syndrome. Other, as yet unidentified, inherited gene mutations are likely. Breast cancer genes can be inherited through both sexes; family members may transmit these genes without developing cancer themselves (that is, penetrance is variable).

Women at risk of familial breast cancer

In the UK, the National Institute for Clinical Excellence has produced clinical guidance for the classification and care of women at risk of familial breast cancer in primary, secondary and tertiary care (Box 5.1). This guidance is presented in terms of where care is likely to be delivered, rather than in categories of risk level, in order to reflect service provision and to try to avoid problems that have been seen previously with the use of low-, medium- and high-risk descriptions.

The optimal screening procedures for women at moderate risk or greater (that is, those who satisfy conditions for referral to secondary or specialist (tertiary) care) have yet to be established. Current recommendations for mammographic surveillance in this group of women are that:

- it should not be available for women younger than 30 years
- it should only be performed as part of a research study or nationally approved and audited service for those aged 30–39 years
- it should be performed annually for women aged 40–49 years
- it should be performed every three years as part of the NHSBSP for women ≥50 years.

Individualized strategies have yet to be developed for women from families with BRCA1, BRCA2 or TP53 mutations.

Ultrasound is not recommended in routine surveillance practice because of a lack of evidence of benefit. Magnetic resonance imaging (MRI) has shown promising results in women at high hereditary risk younger than 50 years. It is more sensitive than mammography (fewer false negatives), but its specificity is lower (more false positives). Importantly, no evidence shows that screening with MRI reduces mortality from breast cancer, and many questions remain unanswered, such as the optimal screening interval and the ages at which screening should start and stop.

The high risk of ovarian cancer associated with carriers of BRCA1 mutations means that annual ovarian screening with transvaginal ultrasound and estimates of levels of CA 125 in serum also are recommended. In the absence of any effective chemoprevention strategies, prophylactic mastectomy is the only option available for preventing breast cancer in known mutation carriers. Although this reduces mortality from breast cancer significantly, it does not completely reduce the risk of breast cancer, as some breast tissue may be left behind. Trials are underway to assess the role of tamoxifen and aromatase inhibitors in the chemoprevention of breast cancer in women at high risk. Breast cancers associated with BRCA1 often do not express hormone receptors, so endocrine chemoprevention may be ineffective.

Counselling and screening must be undertaken only in specialized centres because of the ethical and legal implications. The patient's decision to undergo genetic screening is complicated by the still incomplete understanding of the penetrance of disease in known mutation carriers.

Box 5.1

Clinical guidance for the classification and care of women at risk of familial breast cancer in primary, secondary and tertiary care. Adapted from NICE (2004)

Classification*

- Women at or near population risk (that is, a risk of less than 3% between age 40 and 50 years and a lifetime risk of less than 17%) are cared for in primary care.
- Women at moderate risk (that is, a risk of 3–8% between age 40 and 50 years or a lifetime risk of 17% or greater but less than 30%) are generally cared for in secondary care.
- Women at high risk (that is, a risk of greater than 8% between age 40 and 50 years or a lifetime risk of 30% or greater) are cared for in tertiary care. High risk also includes a 20% or greater chance of a faulty *BRCA1*, *BRCA2* or *TP53* gene in the family.

Referral criteria from primary to secondary care

Women likely to be at moderate risk

- One 1st-degree relative diagnosed before age 40
- One 1st-degree relative and one 2nd degree relative diagnosed after average age 50
- Two 1st-degree relatives diagnosed after average age 50

Women likely to be at more than moderate risk

Female breast cancers only

- One 1st degree relative and one 2nd degree relative diagnosed after average age 50
- Two 1st degree relatives diagnosed after average age 50
- Three or more 1st or 2nd degree relatives diagnosed at any age

Male breast cancer

- One 1st degree male relative diagnosed at any age

Bilateral breast cancer

- One 1st degree relative where 1st primary diagnosed before age 50
- For bilateral breast cancer, each breast has the same count value as one relative

Breast and ovarian cancer

- One 1st or 2nd degree relative with ovarian cancer at any age *and* one 1st or 2nd degree relative with breast cancer at any age (one should be a 1st degree relative)

Referral criteria from secondary to tertiary care

Female breast cancers only
- Two 1st or 2nd degree relatives* diagnosed before average age 50
- Three 1st or 2nd degree relatives* diagnosed before average age 60
- Four relatives† diagnosed at any age

Ovarian cancer
- One relative diagnosed with ovarian cancer at any age *and* on the same side of the family there is
- One 1st (including relative with ovarian cancer) or one 2nd degree relative diagnosed with breast cancer before age 50
- One additional relative diagnosed with ovarian cancer at any age
- Two 1st or 2nd degree relatives diagnosed with breast cancer before average age of 60

Bilateral breast cancer
- One 1st degree relative with cancer diagnosed in both breasts before average age 50
- One 1st or 2nd degree relative diagnosed with bilateral breast cancer *and* one 1st or 2nd degree relative diagnosed with breast cancer before average age 60

Male breast cancer
- One male breast cancer at any age *and* on the same side of the family there is
- One 1st or 2nd degree relative diagnosed with breast cancer before average age 50
- Two 1st or 2nd degree relatives diagnosed with breast cancer before average age 60

*A family history of unusual cancers (bilateral breast cancer, male breast cancer, ovarian cancer, sarcoma at younger than 45 years, glioma or childhood adrenal cortical carcinoma, complicated patterns of multiple cancers at young age) need referral to secondary care.

Women with Jewish ancestry are around 5-10 times more likely to carry BRCA1 and BRCA2 mutations than women in non-Jewish populations.

All relatives must be on the same side of the family and must be blood relatives of the woman and of each other
- 1st degree relative: mother, father, daughter, son, sister, brother
- 2nd degree relative: grandparents, grandchildren, aunt, uncle, niece, nephew, half sister, half brother
- 3rd degree relative: great grandparents, great grandchildren, great aunt, great uncle, first cousin, grand nephew and grand niece.

Women who do not fall into an obvious category can be discussed between primary and secondary, or secondary and tertiary (genetics) care.

†At least one must be a 1st degree relative.

Endometrial assessment

Postmenopausal bleeding and abnormal perimenopausal bleeding are important clinical problems in women who use HRT and those who do not. The main onus is to exclude carcinoma of the endometrium or cervix and premalignant endometrial hyperplasia (Figures 5.1 and 5.2).

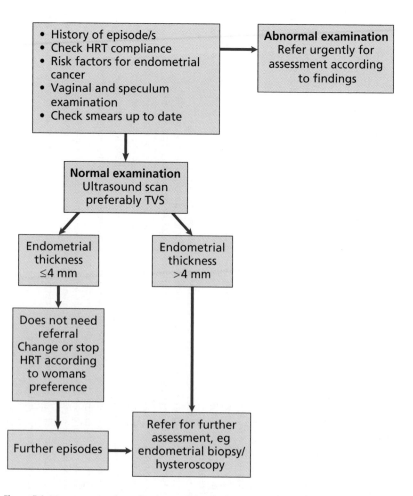

Figure 5.1 Management pathway for abnormal bleeding in women who use HRT. Adapted from Oehler *et al.* (2003). HRT, hormone replacement therapy; TVS, transvaginal ultrasound

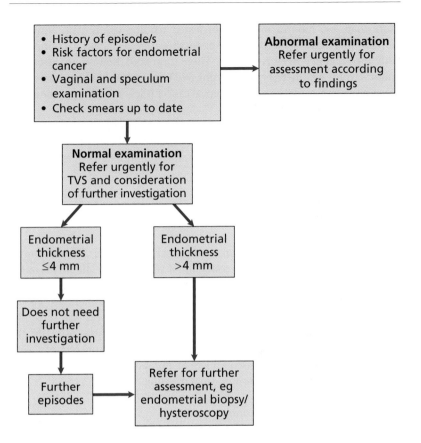

Figure 5.2 Management pathway for abnormal bleeding in women who do not use HRT. Adapted from Oehler *et al.* (2003). TVS, transvaginal ultrasound

When should the endometrium be assessed?

Women who do not use HRT
Abnormal bleeding, such as a postmenopausal bleeding, a sudden change in menstrual pattern, intermenstrual bleeding or postcoital bleeding, requires investigation.

Women who use HRT
With sequential HRT, abnormal bleeding is denoted by a change in pattern of withdrawal bleeds or breakthrough bleeding. In women who take continuous combined or long-cycle regimens, breakthrough bleeding that persists for

more than 4–6 months or does not lessen requires assessment. Similarly, women who have a bleed after amenorrhoea while taking a continuous combined regimen need evaluation. There is no need, however, to assess the endometrium routinely before starting HRT in women with no abnormal bleeding, as the incidence of endometrial cancer is less than one per thousand (<0.1%).

Relevant risk factors for endometrial cancer should be sought in the history. These include nulliparity, late menopause, diabetes, obesity, chronic anovulation use of unopposed oestrogens and a family history of endometrial cancer.

Methods of assessment

Clinical assessment
After a medical history is taken, abdominal and pelvic examination is recommended in all women who complain of abnormal bleeding. This initial assessment should be undertaken in primary care. Cervical cytology should be up to date in accordance with local screening programmes. As an alternative to conventional cervical cytology smear tests, cervical screening may be performed with liquid-based cytology. In women who use HRT, the type of treatment should be documented, as should concordance with treatment – for example, missed tablets or non-adherent patches that may ultimately be implicated in the abnormal bleeding.

Transvaginal ultrasound scanning
Transvaginal ultrasound scanning (TVS) has become a routine procedure for initial assessment. It measures endometrial thickness and also gives information on other pelvic pathology, such as fibroids and ovarian cysts. This technique is less invasive than endometrial biopsy or hysteroscopy but does not give a histological diagnosis. A thickened endometrium or a cavity filled with fluid indicates an increased risk of malignancy or other pathology (hyperplasia or polyps).

Transvaginal ultrasound scanning should be considered as an initial investigation in patients with abnormal uterine bleeding to select those in need of further diagnostic evaluation.

Endometrial thickness cut-off values
Premenopausally, total anteroposterior thickness (both endometrial layers) varies from 4–8 mm in the proliferative phase and peaks at 8–16 mm during the secretory phase. Some debate surrounds whether a 5 mm or 4 mm cut-off value should be used in postmenopausal women who do and do not use HRT: 4 mm may be preferred, as 10-year follow-up data are available. It

must be remembered that endometrial thickness in women who take sequential HRT will vary depending on the phase of therapy (oestrogen alone or oestrogen combined with progestogen). It would be preferable, therefore, to perform TVS after the bleed has ceased and before the combined oestrogen plus progestogen phase is started. In women who take continuous combined regimens, women who use the Mirena coil to provide the progestogen and women who do not use HRT, however, TVS can be performed at any time.

Future developments
Detection of benign lesions, such as endometrial polyps and submucous fibroids, can be enhanced by sonohysterography. By instillation of saline into the uterine cavity, an interface between the fluid and an endometrial mass can be defined more clearly. Some studies suggest that TVS in combination with colour-flow Doppler may help in the diagnosis of endometrial cancer, as blood flow is increased in malignancies. Increased blood flow has also been reported in benign conditions, however, and results are conflicting about whether or not Doppler sonography improves diagnosis of premalignant and malignant endometrial lesions.

Endometrial biopsy
The principal purpose of endometrial biopsy is to diagnose or exclude malignant and premalignant disease (hyperplasia with cytological atypia). Two main techniques are used: aspiration curettage as an outpatient procedure and dilatation and curettage (D&C) under anaesthetic. No existing method will sample the entire uterine cavity. In most cases, therefore, endometrial biopsy has to be complementary to other techniques, such as TVS or hysteroscopy, to increase sensitivity.

The advantage of aspiration curettage is that it avoids general anaesthesia and has fewer complications than D&C, such as bleeding and uterine perforation. A variety of instruments with narrow cannulas for endometrial biopsy have been developed: a commonly used device is the Pipelle. This device obtains an adequate endometrial specimen in up to 99% of women, and a meta-analysis found that it has a detection rate of 99.6% for endometrial carcinoma in postmenopausal women.

Endometrial histology
Proliferative and secretory changes are reported in endometrium removed from normal women. In the case of endometrial hyperplasia, the situation is more complicated, because several classifications have been used over the years. The only important distinction in prognostic and therapeutic terms is between hyperplasias that are associated with a significant risk of progressing

into an endometrial adenocarcinoma and those devoid of such risk. The WHO classification has four categories:

1. Simple hyperplasia
2. Complex hyperplasia
3. Simple atypical hyperplasia
4. Complex atypical hyperplasia.

Only hyperplasia with cytological atypia has significant potential for malignant change. Furthermore, it can co-exist with endometrial cancer. Progression from hyperplasia to cancer has been reported to occur in only 1–3% of patients with hyperplasia without atypia but in 28% of patients with atypical hyperplasia over an average of 13.4 years.

Hysteroscopy

Hysteroscopy allows direct visualization of the uterine cavity. It is known to be a superior method for the detection of endometrial polyps and submucosal myomas, which can easily be missed by endometrial biopsy procedures, ultrasonography or 'blind' curettage. Diagnostic hysteroscopy can be performed as an outpatient procedure without anaesthetic or as a formal theatre procedure.

Hysteroscopy has been advocated by many as the standard for the diagnosis of abnormal uterine bleeding, but it is not 100% accurate and pathology can be missed. A systematic quantitative review found that the diagnostic accuracy of hysteroscopy is high for endometrial cancer but only moderate for non-malignant or premalignant endometrial disease.

In addition, caution is advised in the uncritical use of hysteroscopy in patients suspected of having endometrial cancer, as it could adversely affect prognosis. Hysteroscopy has been shown to cause dissemination of functionally viable malignant cells into the abdominal cavity from uteri that contain endometrial carcinoma, but this is extremely rare, with the literature based solely on case reports.

Bone density estimation

General agreement is that population screening for osteoporosis is not advised. Much can be gained, however, by the selective examination of women from groups at particular risk (Figure 5.3).

Dual energy X-ray absorptiometry

Dual energy X-ray absorptiometry (DXA) is an X-ray based system that uses two different energies to differentiate between soft tissue and bone. The X-rays are directed anterior–posterior or vice versa, depending on the instrument.

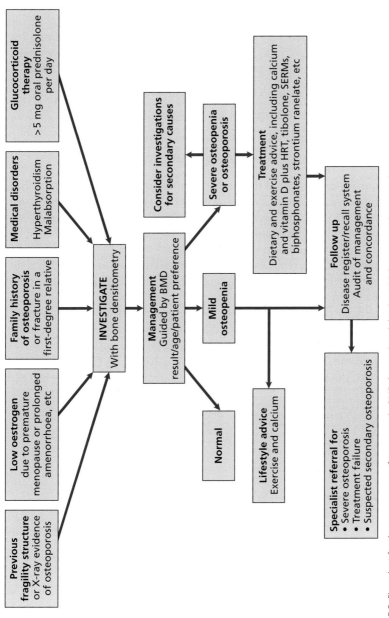

Figure 5.3 Flow chart for the management of osteoporosis. BMD, bone mineral density; HRT, hormone replacement therapy; SERMs, selective (o)estrogen recepor modulators

Fan-beam and pencil-beam machines can scan laterally around the side of a patient, which is useful for measuring the bone density of the lumbar spine.

Values for bone mineral density (BMD) may be quoted as g/cm² or converted into values that relate to the average young normal female (or male) peak bone mass or to the bone mass related to the patient's age group. These are T scores and Z scores, respectively, and are calculated as follows:

- T score = $\dfrac{\text{Patient's BMD–population peak BMD}}{\text{Standard deviation (SD) of population peak BMD}}$

- Z score = $\dfrac{\text{Patient's BMD–population age-related BMD}}{\text{SD of population age-related BMD}}$

In women, peak density of the lumbar spine is reached around the middle of the third decade of life. According to WHO (1994), osteoporosis is diagnosed if the T score is –2.5 or lower (see Chapter 3).

Values can be plotted on a chart to show the mean and limits of +2 or –2 SD of a healthy population (Figure 5.4).

Calibrations for average bone densities often are based on a US database of the upper femur, called the National Health and Nutrition Examination Survey (NHANES) database.

The main sites for measurement are the spine (L1 or L2–L4) and various regions of interest at the hip. Some difficulties are encountered in measuring the spine. This occurs especially in the elderly where osteophytes due to osteoarthritis, kyphosis, scoliosis and aortic calcification can lead to falsely increased values of BMD. It is now recommended, therefore, that the best site

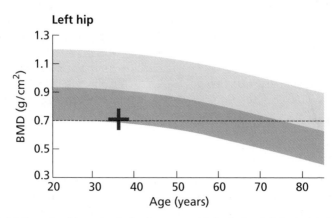

Figure 5.4 Femoral neck bone density showing mean and limits of +2 and –2 standard deviations of a healthy population

to measure for diagnosis is the hip. Bone mineral density of the 'total hip' and the neck of femur are the most commonly used measurements.

Peripheral DXA (pDXA) systems are also now available to measure the forearm or calcaneus and may be considered to be a risk assessment tool. They cannot replace hip DXA, however, for the formal diagnosis of osteoporosis.

Generally agreed indications for densitometry are:

- Any oestrogen-deficient postmenopausal woman who would want to be treated or would want to continue treatment if found to be osteopenic or osteoporotic.
- Patients older than 50 years suspected to be osteoporotic on X-ray or clinically through height loss or low impact fracture, such as Colles' radial fracture or fracture of any peripheral bone excluding the digits.
- Patients who have a medical condition that predisposes to osteoporosis if effective treatment is available – for example, metabolic bone disease, thyroid disease, liver disease, anorexia nervosa, malabsorption syndromes and other rarer causes of osteoporosis.
- Patients who use systemic corticosteroids with a daily dose >5 mg prednisolone or equivalent for a projected duration of three months or longer.
- Oestrogen-deficient women younger than 45 years who experience primary amenorrhoea or secondary amenorrhoea (including that resulting from hysterectomy).
- Patients with a history of fracture, particularly hip fracture, in a first-degree relative.

The frequency of follow-up scans for those at risk of osteoporosis or those being treated for established disease is controversial. Initially, follow-up scans may be undertaken at two years to assess response to treatment and, in general, should not be done more frequently than every three years thereafter. When BMD is measured by densitometry, atom for atom, strontium attenuates X-rays more strongly than calcium, as it has a higher atomic number (calcium 20, strontium 38), which can lead to an overestimation of the BMD value. The use of bone markers, in the future, however, may replace DXA for early assessment of response to treatment.

Quantitative ultrasound

This technique involves the transmission of a low-amplitude ultrasound beam, usually through the calcaneus, and measures bone strength. It has the attraction of being portable and not using ionizing radiation. It remains to be evaluated fully before it can be used in routine clinical practice. In terms of diagnostic capability, most data involve prediction of fractures in elderly women, in whom it seems to be a competent measure of the risk of hip fracture. It remains to be determined, however, whether it can predict fracture at other sites or in younger menopausal women.

Single energy X-ray absorptiometry

This method is used commonly for wrist scans.

Quantitative computed tomography

This provides measurement of the spine, hip and wrist. It does not have a diagnostic ability superior to that of DXA. Its use in clinical practice is limited by poorer precision and much higher radiation doses than used with DXA.

Biochemical markers of bone metabolism

Over the last decade, our ability to detect the subtle changes in bone turnover associated with postmenopausal bone loss and osteoporosis has been enhanced by the development of specific and sensitive markers of this process.

Table 5.1

Most commonly used biochemical markers of bone turnover. Adapted from Hannon and Eastell (2003)

Bone formation	Bone resorption
By-products of collagen synthesis	Collagen degradation products
• Pro-collagen type 1 C terminal pro-peptide (PICP)*	• Hydroxyproline (Hyp)†
• Pro-collagen type 1 N terminal pro-peptide (PINP)*	• Pyridinoline (PYD)*†
Matrix protein	• Deoxypyridinoline (DPD)*†
• Osteocalcin (OC)*	Crosslinked telopeptides of type I collagen
Osteoblast enzyme	• N-terminal crosslinked telopeptide (NTX)*†
• Total alkaline phosphatase (total ALP)*	• C-terminal crosslinked telopeptide (CTX)*†
• Bone alkaline phosphatase (bone ALP)*	• C-terminal crosslinked telopeptide generated by matrix metalloproteinases (MMPs) (CTX-MMP, formerly ICTP)*
	Osteoclast enzyme
	• Tartrate-resistant acid phosphatase (TRACP)*

*Measured in serum
†Measured in urine

Biochemical markers of bone turnover are classified as markers of resorption or formation. It should be remembered, however, that bone resorption and formation are 'coupled' processes, and, therefore, in most situations, any marker can be used to determine the overall rate of bone turnover. Most markers of bone resorption are products of collagen degradation that are released into the circulation and finally excreted in the urine. Tartrate-resistant acid phosphatase is secreted by osteoclasts and levels are measured in serum.

Markers of bone formation are by-products of collagen formation, matrix proteins or enzymes associated with osteoblast activity (Table 5.1). A potential use of these markers is to monitor anti-osteoporotic therapy, as they will show changes within 3–6 months, while DXA will take more than one year. These markers, however, have not yet been evaluated fully for routine use.

Further reading

Endocrine

Davis SR, Davison SK, Donath S, et al. Circulating androgen levels and self-reported sexual function in women. *JAMA* 2005;**294**:91–6.

Parker S. Follicle stimulating hormone: facts and fallacies. *J Br Menopause Soc* 2004;**10**:166–8.

Slater CC, Hodis HN, Mack WJ, et al. Markedly elevated levels of estrone sulfate after long-term oral, but not transdermal, administration of estradiol in postmenopausal women. *Menopause* 2001;**8**:200–3.

Mammography and genetic screening

Aiello EJ, Buist DS, White E, Porter PL. Association between mammographic breast density and breast cancer tumor characteristics. *Cancer Epidemiol Biomarkers Prev* 2005;**14**:662–8.

Ames JE, Trute L, White D, et al. Distinct molecular pathogenesis of early-onset breast cancers in BRCA1 and BRCA 2 mutation carriers: population based study. *Cancer Res* 1999;**59**:2011–17.

Anderson G. *Part I: Statistical Issues in WHI. Part II: Further Analyses of Prior Hormone Therapy on Breast Cancer. The WHI Estrogen + Progestin Trial.* Seattle, WA: Fred Hutchinson Cancer Research Center, 2003. www.fda.gov/ohrms/dockets/ac/03/slides/3992S1_05_Anderson.ppt (last accessed 29 September 2005).

Banks E, Reeves G, Beral V, et al. Impact of use of hormone replacement therapy on false positive recall in the NHS breast screening programme: results from the Million Women Study. *BMJ* 2004;**328**:1291–2.

Blanks RG, Wallis MG, Moss SM. A comparison of cancer detection rates achieved by breast cancer screening programmes by number of readers, for one and two view mammography: results from the UK National Health Service breast screening programme. *J Med Screen* 1998;**5**:195–201.

Chlebowski RT, Hendrix SL, Langer RD, *et al*. Influence of estrogen plus progestin on breast cancer and mammography in healthy postmenopausal women. The Women's Health Initiative randomized trial. *JAMA* 2003;**289**:3243–53.

Claus EB, Schildkraut JM, Thompson WD, Risch NJ. The genetic attributable risk of breast and ovarian cancer. *Cancer* 1996;**77**:2318–24.

Colacurci N, Fornaro F, De Franciscis P, *et al*. Effects of a short-term suspension of hormone replacement therapy on mammographic density. *Fertil Steril* 2001;**76**:451–5.

Cuzick J, Powles T, Veronesi U, *et al*. Overview of the main outcomes in breast-cancer prevention trials. *Lancet* 2003;**361**:296–300.

Daling JR, Malone KE, Doody DR, *et al*. Association of regimens of hormone replacement therapy to prognostic factors among women diagnosed with breast cancer aged 50–64 years. *Cancer Epidemiol Biomarkers Prev* 2003;**12**:1175–81.

Greendale GA, Reboussin BA, Sie A, *et al*. Effects of estrogen and estrogen-progestin on mammographic parenchymal density. Postmenopausal Estrogen/Progestin Interventions (PEPI) Investigators. *Ann Intern Med* 1999;**130**:262–9.

Greendale GA, Reboussin BA, Slone S, *et al*. Postmenopausal hormone therapy and change in mammographic density. *J Natl Cancer Inst* 2003;**95**:30–7.

Harvey JA, Bovbjerg VE. Quantitative assessment of mammographic breast density: relationship with breast cancer risk. *Radiology* 2004;**230**:29–41.

Harvey JA, Pinkerton JV, Herman CR. Short-term cessation of hormone replacement therapy and improvement of mammographic specificity. *J Natl Cancer Inst* 1997;**89**:1623–5.

Kerlikowske K, Shepherd J, Creasman J, *et al*. Are breast density and bone mineral density independent risk factors for breast cancer? *J Natl Cancer Inst* 2005;**97**:368–74.

Lichtenstein P, Holm N, Verkasalo P, *et al*. Environmental and heritable factors in the causation of cancer – analyses of cohorts of twins from Sweden, Denmark, and Finland. *N Engl J Med* 2000;**343**:78–85.

MARIBS study group. Screening with magnetic resonance imaging and mammography of a UK population at high familial risk of breast cancer: a prospective multicentre cohort study (MARIBS). *Lancet* 2005;**365**:1769–78.

McTiernan A, Martin CF, Peck JD, *et al*; Women's Health Initiative Mammogram Density Study Investigators. Estrogen-plus-progestin use and mammographic density in postmenopausal women: women's health initiative randomized trial. *J Natl Cancer Inst* 2005;**97**:1366–76.

Narod SA, Brunet JS, Ghadirian P, *et al*. Tamoxifen and risk of contralateral breast cancer in BRCA1 and BRCA2 mutation carriers: a case control study. *Lancet* 2000;**356**:1876–81.

Nathanson KN, Wooster R, Weber BL. Breast cancer genetics: what we know and what we need. *Nature Med* 2001;**7**:552–6.

National Institute for Clinical Excellence. *Clinical Guidelines for the Classification and Care of Women At Risk of Familial Breast Cancer in Primary, Secondary and Tertiary Care*. London: NICE, 2004. Available at: http://www.nice.org.uk/ (last accessed 29 September 2005).

Rutter CM, Mandelson MT, Laya MB, *et al*. Changes in breast density associated with initiation, discontinuation, and continuing use of hormone replacement therapy. *JAMA* 2001;**285**:171–6.

Stallard S, Litherland JC, Cordiner CM, *et al.* Effect of hormone replacement therapy on the pathological stage of breast cancer: population based cross-sectional study. *BMJ* 2000;**320**:348–9.

Sterns EE, Zee B. Mammographic density changes in perimenopausal and postmenopausal women: is effect of hormone replacement therapy predictable? *Breast Cancer Res Treat* 2000;**59**:125–32.

Szabo CL, King M. Population genetics of BRCA1 and BRCA2. *Am J Hum Genet* 1997;**60**:1013–20.

Warner E, Causer PA. MRI surveillance for hereditary breast-cancer risk. *Lancet* 2005;**365**:1747–9

Warren R. Hormones and mammographic breast density. *Maturitas* 2004;**49**:67–78.

Endometrial assessment

Affinito P, Palomba S, Sammartino A, *et al.* Ultrasonographic endometrial monitoring during continuous-sequential hormonal replacement therapy regimen in postmenopausal women. *Maturitas* 2001;**39**:239–44.

Arikan G, Reich O, Weiss U, *et al.* Are endometrial carcinoma cells disseminated at hysteroscopy functionally viable? *Gynecol Oncol* 2001;**83**:221–6.

Ballester MJ, Girones R, Torres JV, *et al.* Diagnosis of endometrial carcinoma: predictive value of transvaginal color Doppler. *J Gynecol Surg* 1994;**10**:173–83.

Bergman L, Beelen M, Gallee M, *et al.* Risk and prognosis of endometrial cancer after tamoxifen for breast cancer. *Lancet* 2000;**356**:881–7.

Clark TJ, Voit D, Gupta JK, *et al.* Accuracy of hysteroscopy in the diagnosis of endometrial cancer and hyperplasia: a systematic quantitative review. *JAMA* 2002;**288**:1610–21.

Dijkhuizen FP, Mol BW, Brolmann HA, Heintz AP. The accuracy of endometrial sampling in the diagnosis of patients with endometrial carcinoma and hyperplasia: a meta-analysis. *Cancer* 2000;**89**:1765–72.

Epstein E, Ramirez A, Skoog L, Valentin L. Dilatation and curettage fails to detect most focal lesions in the uterine cavity in women with postmenopausal bleeding. *Acta Obstet Gynecol Scand* 2001;**80**:1131–6.

Epstein E, Ramirez A, Skoog L, Valentin L. Transvaginal sonography, saline contrast sonohysterography and hysteroscopy for the investigation of women with postmenopausal bleeding and endometrium >5 mm. *Ultrasound Obstet Gynecol* 2001;**18**:157–62.

Gull B, Karlsson B, Milsom I, Granberg S. Can ultrasound replace dilatation and curettage? A longitudinal evaluation of postmenopausal bleeding and transvaginal sonographic measurement of the endometrium as predictors of endometrial cancer. *Am J Obstet Gynecol* 2003;**188**:401–8.

Gupta JK, Chien PF, Voit D, *et al.* Ultrasonographic endometrial thickness for diagnosing endometrial pathology in women with postmenopausal bleeding: a meta-analysis. *Acta Obstet Gynecol Scand* 2002;**81**:799–816.

Kurman RJ, Kaminski PF, Norris HJ. The behavior of endometrial hyperplasia. A long-term study of 'untreated' hyperplasia in 170 patients. *Cancer* 1985;**56**:403–12.

Medverd JR, Dubinsky TJ. Cost analysis model: US versus endometrial biopsy in evaluation of peri- and postmenopausal abnormal vaginal bleeding. *Radiology* 2002;**222**:619–27.

Oehler MK, MacKenzie I, Kehoe S, Rees MCP. Assessment of abnormal bleeding in menopausal women: an update. *J Br Menopause Soc* 2003; **9**: 117–22.

NHS Cancer Screening Programmes. *NHS Cervical Screening Programme.* Sheffield: NHS Cancer Screening Programmes. Available at: www.cancerscreening.org.uk/cervical (last accessed 29 September 2005).

Sankaranarayanan R, Gaffikin L, Jacob M, *et al*. A critical assessment of screening methods for cervical neoplasia. *Int J Gynaecol Obstet* 2005;**89**(Suppl 2):S4–12.

Smith-Bindman R, Kerlikowske K, Feldstein VA, *et al*. Endovaginal ultrasound to exclude endometrial cancer and other endometrial abnormalities. *JAMA* 1998;**280**:1510–17.

Weiderpass E, Persson I, Adami HO, *et al*. Body size in different periods of life, diabetes mellitus, hypertension, and risk of postmenopausal endometrial cancer (Sweden). *Cancer Causes Control* 2000;**11**:185–92.

Bone

Berger A. Bone mineral density scans. *BMJ* 2002;**325**:484.

Chen P, Satterwhite JH, Licata AA, *et al*. Early changes in biochemical markers of bone formation predict BMD response to teriparatide in postmenopausal women with osteoporosis. *J Bone Miner Res* 2005;**20**:962–70.

Cook RB, Collins D, Tucker J, Zioupos P. Comparison of questionnaire and quantitative ultrasound techniques as screening tools for DXA. *Osteoporos Int* 2005;May 10; [Epub ahead of print].

Hannon RA, Eastell R. Biochemical markers of bone turnover and fracture prediction. *J Br Menopause Soc* 2003;**9**:10–15.

Hodson J, Marsh J. Quantitative ultrasound and risk factor enquiry as predictors of postmenopausal osteoporosis: comparative study in primary care. *BMJ* 2003;**326**:1250–1.

Looker AC, Wahner HW, Dunn WL, *et al*. Updated data on proximal femur bone mineral levels of US adults. *Osteoporos Int* 1998;**8**:468–89.

Osteoporosis prevention, diagnosis, and therapy. *NIH Consensus Statement* 2000;**17**:1–45.

World Health Organization. *Assessment of Fracture Risk and its Application to Screening for Postmenopausal Osteoporosis. WHO Technical Report Series 843.* Geneva: WHO, 1994.

MANAGEMENT STRATEGIES

6 Oestrogen-based hormone replacement therapy

At present, more than 50 hormone replacement therapy (HRT) preparations, which feature different strengths, combinations and routes of administration, are licensed in the UK. The very title of 'HRT' may change in the future to ET (estrogen therapy) for oestrogen therapy and EPT (estrogen and progestogen therapy) for combined preparations – whether sequential or continuous combined.

Components of hormone replacement therapy

Hormone replacement therapy consists of an oestrogen combined with a progestogen in non-hysterectomized women. Progestogens are given cyclically or continuously with the oestrogen. Different routes of administration are employed: oral, transdermal, subcutaneous, intranasal and vaginal.

Oestrogens

Two types of oestrogen are available: synthetic and natural. Synthetic oestrogens, such as ethinyl oestradiol and mestranol, are generally considered to be not suitable for HRT because of their greater metabolic impact. Natural oestrogens include oestradiol, oestrone and oestriol, which, although chemically synthesized from soya beans or yams, are molecularly identical to the natural human hormone. Conjugated equine oestrogens contain about 50–65% oestrone sulphate, and the remainder consists of equine oestrogens – mainly equilin sulphate. These may also be classified as 'natural'. Much confusion surrounds what constitutes a 'natural' oestrogen. In this book, we have taken the view that a 'natural' oestrogen is one that is found in normal physiology irrespective of whether it has been prepared by chemical synthesis or extraction from a plant or animal source.

The generally accepted minimum bone-sparing doses of oestrogen are listed below (Table 6.1), although increasing evidence shows that even lower doses may be effective. Although these may also improve vasomotor symptoms, oestrogenic side-effects may be reduced. Young women who experience a surgical menopause, however, initially may need higher doses of oestrogen to alleviate menopausal symptoms. Conversely, older women usually require lower doses to control their symptoms.

Table 6.1

Minimum bone-sparing doses of HRT

HRT	Dose
Oestradiol oral	1–2 mg
Oestradiol patch	25–50 µg
Oestradiol gel	1–5 g*
Oestradiol implant	50 mg every six months
Conjugated equine oestrogens	0.3–0.625 mg daily

*Depends on preparation

Progestogens

The progestogens used in HRT are almost all synthetic, are structurally different to progesterone and are also derived from plant sources. Currently, they are used mainly in tablet form, although norethisterone and levonorgestrel are available in transdermal patches combined with oestradiol, and levonorgestrel can be delivered directly to the uterus (Table 6.2). The native molecule progesterone is formulated as a 4% vaginal gel and is licensed for use in HRT, but its availability varies worldwide. A progesterone pessary to be used vaginally or rectally is available, but this is currently not licensed for HRT.

The synthetic progestogens studied so far in HRT are derived from progesterone (17-hydroxyprogesterone derivatives and 19-norprogesterone

Table 6.2

Acceptable regimens of progestogen for endometrial protection.* Source: MIMS, British National Formulary (2005)

HRT	Regimen	
	Dose	Timing of dose
Sequential		
Dydrogesterone oral	10–20 mg	Last 14 days of a 28-day cycle
Levonorgestrel oral	75–250 µg	Last 10–12 days of a 28-day cycle
Levonorgestrel patch	10 µg	Last 14 days of a 28-day cycle
Medroxyprogesterone acetate oral	10 mg	Last 14 days of a 28-day cycle
	20 mg	Last 14 days of a three-month cycle
Norethisterone oral	1 mg	Last 10–14 days of a 28-day cycle
Norethisterone patch	170 µg or 250 µg	Last 14 days of a 28-day cycle
Norgestrel oral	150–500 µg	Last 10–12 days of a 28-day cycle
Progesterone vaginal	4% gel	Alternate days for last 12 days of 28-day cycle
Continuous		
Drospirenone oral	2 mg	Daily
Dydrogesterone oral	5 mg	Daily
Levonorgestrel patch	7 µg	Daily
Medroxyprogesterone acetate oral	2.5–5.0 mg	Daily
Norethisterone oral	0.5–1 mg	Daily
Norethisterone patch	170 µg	Daily

*Depends on preparation

derivatives) or testosterone (19-nortestosterone derivatives). The 17-hydroxyprogesterone and 19-nortestosterone derivatives are the progestogens used most commonly in HRT.

1. 17-hydroxyprogesterone derivatives: dydrogesterone, medroxyprogesterone acetate
2. 19-nortestosterone derivatives: the estrane group includes norethisterone, and the gonane group includes levonorgestrel and its derivatives, such as, desogestrel, etonorgestrel and norgestimate, which have been referred to as third-generation progestogens.

Several new progestogens have been synthesized in the last decade and may be considered as fourth-generation progestogens. Dienogest is referred to as a hybrid progestogen, as it is derived from the estrane group with a 17α-cyanomethyl group, and drospirenone is derived from spirolactone. These two progestogens have a partial anti-androgenic effect. Drospirenone also has anti-mineralocorticoid properties. The 9-norprogesterone derivatives, trimegestone and nomegestrol acetate, have also been studied in HRT regimens.

Tibolone

Tibolone is a synthetic steroid compound that is itself inert, but, on absorption, it is converted *in vivo* to metabolites with oestrogenic, progestogenic and androgenic actions. It is used in postmenopausal women who wish to have amenorrhoea. It is classified as HRT in the *British National Formulary*. It is used to treat vasomotor, psychological and libido problems. The daily dose is 2.5 mg. It conserves bone mass, and fracture data are awaited.

Androgens

Testosterone implants may be used to improve libido but are not successful in all women, as other factors, such as marital problems, may be involved. Testosterone patches and gels are currently licensed for use in men and are being evaluated intensively in clinical trials for potential use in women who complain of low libido.

Delivery systems

Oral versus parenteral administration

The main consideration in route of administration is whether to use oral or non-oral delivery. The latter avoids the gut and first-pass effects on the liver. After oral administration, the dominant circulating oestrogen is oestrone, while after parenteral administration it is oestradiol.

Substances normally synthesized in the liver may be affected differentially by oral or parenteral delivery. For example, high doses of conjugated equine oestrogens increase the production of renin substrate, but the type of substrate induced is not the one normally associated with hypertension. The clinical significance is unclear, as blood pressure does not normally increase with this form of HRT. Oral oestrogen also induces the hepatic production and release of sex hormone binding globulin. Furthermore, production of certain coagulation factors and lipids may be affected differentially by the route of administration.

Extensive debate currently surrounds the relative merits of the oral route versus the non-oral route. At present, the transdermal route seems to have no clear advantage over the oral route. Furthermore, all oestrogens, regardless of the route of administration, eventually pass through the liver and are recycled by the enterohepatic circulation. In routine clinical practice, therefore, the oral route is the usual first line of treatment unless the patient has a pre-existing medical condition. Some practitioners, however, prefer to embark on transdermal treatment on the grounds that it mimics the natural route of oestrogen delivery in premenopausal women – when oestrogen is delivered from the ovaries directly into the venous system.

Non-oral delivery systems

Transdermal systems: patch and gel
Oestradiol and progestogens can diffuse through the skin. Two transdermal systems are available: patch and gel. Two patch technologies exist: alcohol-based reservoir patches, which have an adhesive outer ring, and matrix patches, in which the hormone is distributed evenly throughout the adhesive. Skin reactions are less common with matrix patches than with reservoir patches. Of the progestogens, currently only norethisterone and levonorgestrel are delivered transdermally in patches. At present, only oestradiol is delivered in a gel.

Implants
Oestradiol implants are crystalline pellets of oestradiol that are inserted subcutaneously under local anaesthetic and release oestradiol over many months. Implants have the advantage that once inserted patients do not have to remember to take their drugs. A significant concern is tachyphylaxis, which may be defined as a recurrence of menopausal symptoms while the implant is still releasing adequate levels of oestradiol. Another concern is that implants may remain effective for many years. A check on levels of oestradiol in plasma before re-implantation should be considered, especially in women who return more frequently for treatment, to ensure that the pre-implantation level is in the normal premenopausal range (<1000 pmol/l).

Nasal spray
Oestradiol can be delivered by nasal spray. After intranasal dosing, oestradiol is absorbed rapidly, with plasma concentrations reaching maximal values after 10–30 minutes and returning to levels of untreated postmenopausal women within 12 hours. Further intranasal administration of 300 µg/day oestradiol seems to be as effective in alleviating postmenopausal symptoms as oral administration of 2 mg/day oestradiol.

Vaginal ring
Systemic delivery of oestradiol can also be achieved with vaginal rings.

Intrauterine systems
Originally used to provide contraception, the intrauterine system delivers 20 µg/day of levonorgestrel to the endometrium and can provide the

progestogen component of HRT. The oestrogen can then be given orally or transdermally. This system also provides a solution to the problem of contraception in the perimenopause and is also the only way in which a 'no bleed' regimen can be achieved in perimenopausal women. A device that releases 10 µg/day is being evaluated for early postmenopausal women.

Hysterectomized women

About 20% of women in the UK have been estimated to have undergone hysterectomy by the age of 52 years. In general, hysterectomized women should be given oestrogen alone and have no need for a progestogen. Furthermore, combined HRT may confer a greater risk of breast cancer than oestrogen alone (see Chapter 7). Concern about a remnant of endometrium in the cervical stump may exist in women who have had a subtotal hysterectomy. If this is suspected to be the case, the presence or absence of bleeding induced by monthly sequential HRT may be a useful diagnostic test.

Non-hysterectomized women

Progestogens are added to oestrogens to reduce the increased risk of endometrial hyperplasia and carcinoma, which occurs with unopposed oestrogen; they need not be given to women who have undergone hysterectomy. Progestogen can be given 'sequentially' for 10–14 days every four weeks, for 14 days every 13 weeks or every day – that is, 'continuously'. The first leads to monthly bleeds, the second to bleeds every three months and the last aims to achieve amenorrhoea. Progestogen must be given to women who have undergone endometrial ablative techniques, as it cannot be assumed that all the endometrium has been removed – even if prolonged amenorrhoea has been achieved.

Perimenopausal women

The options available are monthly cyclic or three-monthly cyclic regimens. For women with infrequent menstruation and those who are intolerant of progestogens, a three-monthly preparation can be considered. Only one is available in the UK at present: it contains oestradiol valerate and medroxyprogesterone acetate. Continuous combined regimens should not be used in perimenopausal women because of the high risk of irregular bleeding.

Postmenopausal women

By strict definition, women are considered to be postmenopausal 12 months after their last menstrual period. In clinical practice, however, the definition is difficult to apply, especially in women who started HRT in the perimenopause. Although monthly and three-monthly cyclic or continuous combined regimens can be used in postmenopausal women, the last are more popular because of the lack of induced bleeding. Furthermore, continuous combined treatment may have a reduced risk of endometrial cancer compared with sequential regimens (see Chapter 7). Continuous combined therapy induces endometrial atrophy.

Irregular bleeding or spotting can occur during the first 4–6 months of continuous combined therapy and does not warrant investigation. Endometrial assessment needs to be considered if the bleeding becomes heavier rather than lighter, if it persists beyond six months or if it occurs after a significant time of amenorrhoea (see Chapter 4). The incidence of irregular bleeding may be reduced by increasing the ratio of the progestogen to the oestrogen.

Switching from sequential to continuous combined therapy

It may be difficult to decide when women can switch over from sequential to continuous combined therapy. Pragmatically, postmenopausal status can be estimated from:

- **age:** it has been estimated that 80% of women will be postmenopausal by the age of 54 years
- **previous amenorrhoea or increased levels of follicle-stimulating hormone (FSH):** women who experienced six months of amenorrhoea or had increased levels of FSH in their mid 40s are likely to be post-menopausal after taking several years of monthly sequential HRT.

Starting systemic HRT

Symptoms of oestrogen deficiency, such as hot flushes, mood changes, tiredness, arthralgia and vaginal dryness, may start several months or years before periods stop: such a history in women older than 40 years is a classic presentation. Amenorrhoea need not be awaited before HRT is started. The dose used should control the individual's menopausal symptoms, and control of symptoms could be considered to be a 'barometer' of the minimum required dose.

Managing the side-effects of systemic HRT

Side-effects can be related to oestrogen or progestogen, or a combination of both. Many of the so-called 'side-effects' of HRT, in fact, are start-up effects consequent to administration of oestrogen, which previously had been lacking. Furthermore, side-effects are more likely to be problematic in women who have been deficient in oestrogen for a long period. It is essential, therefore, to discuss early effects, such as breast tenderness, at the outset and to explain that they usually resolve by three months into treatment. If unprepared for start-up effects women will be alarmed and may well stop the HRT. Usually, it is possible to determine whether the side-effects are oestrogenic (occurring continuously or randomly throughout the cycle) or progestogenic (occurring in a cyclical pattern during the progestogen phase of sequential HRT).

Side-effects

Oestrogen-related side-effects include fluid retention, bloating, breast tenderness or enlargement, nausea, headaches, leg cramps and dyspepsia.

Progestogen-related side-effects are fluid retention, breast tenderness, headaches or migraine, mood swings, depression, acne, lower abdominal pain and backache.

Complaints of weight gain and poor cycle control are common to both elements.

Management strategies

Management strategies that are useful in clinical practice will be described; interestingly, none have been examined systematically in clinical trials.

Oestrogen-related side-effects

Transient side-effects
Side-effects are often transient and resolve without any change in treatment with increasing duration of use. Patients should be encouraged to persist with therapy for about 12 weeks to await resolution. The analogy with certain symptoms of early pregnancy may be useful. Patients can be reassured and given appropriate advice in order to minimize these problems.

Breast tenderness may be alleviated with addition of gamolenic acid. Leg cramps can improve with lifestyle changes. Nausea or gastric upset with oral preparations may be alleviated by adjusting the timing of the dose or taking the dose with food; lactose sensitivity should be considered.

Persistent side-effects
With persistent side-effects, the options include:

- **reduce dose** – when doing this, the endpoints of treatment, such as symptom control and the prevention of osteoporosis, must be borne in mind
- **change oestrogen type** – oestradiol or conjugated equine oestrogens

- **change route of delivery** – oral, patch, gel, nasal spray, vaginal ring or implant.

Progestogen-related side-effects

Progestogenic side-effects are more problematic because of the need to provide endometrial protection. They are connected to type, duration and dose of progestogen. Once again, perseverance with therapy should be encouraged, as hysterectomy must be considered only as a last resort. Useful strategies include:

- change type of progestogen – for example, from a 19-nortestosterone to a 17-hydroxyprogesterone derivative
- reduce dose, but not below the recommended levels for endometrial protection
- change administration route, using transdermal, vaginal or intrauterine progesterone or progestogen
- reduce duration, as progestogens can be taken for 10–14 days of each monthly sequential regimen
- reduce frequency, using long-cycle HRT that administers progestogen for 14 days every three months (but this is suitable only for women without natural regular cycles).

Continuous combined therapy often reduces progestogenic side-effects with established use, but it is suitable only for postmenopausal women.

Weight gain

Weight gain is often given as a major reason why women are reluctant to start or continue treatment. Randomized placebo-controlled trials, however, repeatedly show no evidence of HRT-induced weight gain.

Bleeding

Monthly sequential regimens should produce regular predictable and acceptable bleeding starting towards the end or soon after the end of the progestogen phase. Non-concordance with therapy, drug interactions (including with herbal remedies) or gastrointestinal upset, which can interfere with absorption, need to be excluded. Pelvic pathology will need exclusion if the problem persists or does not respond to treatment (see Chapter 5). Useful strategies include:

- increase dose or change type of progestogen in women with heavy or prolonged bleeding
- increase dose or change type of progestogen in women with bleeding early in the progestogen phase

- change type of progestogen in women with painful bleeding
- change regimen or increase progestogen in women with irregular bleeding.

No bleeding reflects an atrophic endometrium and occurs in 5% of women, but pregnancy needs to be excluded in perimenopausal women. Breakthrough bleeding is common in the first 3–6 months of continuous combined and long-cycle HRT regimens, but if it continues thereafter, it should be investigated as for postmenopausal bleeding (see Chapter 5).

Duration of systemic therapy

The duration of systemic therapy depends on the endpoints of treatment.

Treatment of vasomotor symptoms

Treatment for vasomotor symptoms should be continued for up to five years and then stopped to evaluate whether or not they have recurred. This duration will not significantly increase the risk of breast cancer (see Chapter 7). Although menopausal symptoms usually resolve within 2–5 years, some women experience symptoms for many years – even into their 70s and 80s (see Chapter 2)

Prevention or treatment of osteoporosis

For this issue, treatment needs to be continued for life, as bone mineral density falls when treatment is stopped. Use of HRT for 5–10 years after the menopause has been assumed to delay the peak incidence of hip fracture by a corresponding amount. If the median age of hip fracture is 79 years, therefore, and if this is delayed by 5–10 years through the use of HRT, most women would not live long enough to suffer a hip fracture. Most epidemiological evidence, however, suggests that 5–10 years of HRT soon after the menopause does not give any significant reduction in the risk of hip fracture 30 years later (see Chapter 7). Although some women will be happy to take HRT for life, others may view treatment as a continuum of options and will wish to change to other agents such as raloxifene, a bisphosphonate or strontium ranelate, because of the small but measurable increase in risk of breast cancer associated with the long-term use of combined HRT.

Premature menopause

In this case, women are usually advised to continue with HRT until the average age of the natural menopause – that is 52 years (see Chapter 11). Thereafter, the issues discussed in the above sections are relevant.

Stopping systemic hormone replacement therapy

Various strategies are used, but they have not been examined in clinical trials. The limited evidence available shows no clear advantage of stopping gradually or abruptly. The main issue is a recurrence of menopausal symptoms, such as flushes and myalgia, on stopping, as has been reported by participants of the Women's Health Initiative, who discontinued HRT suddenly. Anecdotally, older women need less oestrogen to control their symptoms and thus a lower dose can be tried before stopping. Although alternate-day, or even less frequent, oral treatment can be used in hysterectomized women, concerns exist that this strategy could lead to irregular bleeding or insufficient addition of progestogen in women whose uterus is intact.

Treatment of local symptoms

Some women do not wish to take, or cannot tolerate, systemic HRT and simply require relief of local symptoms, which usually are urogenital. Synthetic or conjugated equine oestrogens should be avoided, as they are well absorbed from the vagina. The options available are low-dose natural oestrogens, such as vaginal oestriol by cream or pessary or oestradiol by tablet or ring. Treatment is needed long term, if not lifelong, as symptoms return on cessation of treatment. With the recommended dose regimens, no adverse endometrial effects should be incurred, and a progestogen need not be added for endometrial protection with such low-dose preparations.

Further reading

Baracat EC, Barbosa IC, Giordano MG, *et al.* A randomized, open-label study of conjugated equine estrogens plus medroxyprogesterone acetate versus tibolone: effects on symptom control, bleeding pattern, lipid profile and tolerability. *Climacteric* 2002;5:60–9.

Beardsworth SA, Kearney CE, Purdie DW. Prevention of postmenopausal bone loss at lumbar spine and upper femur with tibolone: a two-year randomised controlled trial. *Br J Obstet Gynaecol* 1999;106:678–83.

British Medical Association, Royal Pharmaceutical Society of Great Britain. *British National Formulary*. London: BMA, RPS, 2005. Available at: http://www.bnf.org/bnf/ (last accessed 29 September 2005).

Buckler H, Al-Azzawi F; UK VR Multicentre Trial Group. The effect of a novel vaginal ring delivering oestradiol acetate on climacteric symptoms in postmenopausal women. *BJOG* 2003;110:753–9.

Davis SR. The use of testosterone after menopause. *J Br Menopause Soc* 2004;10:65-9.

Delmas PD, Marianowski L, Perez Ade C, *et al.* Prevention of postmenopausal bone loss by pulsed estrogen therapy: comparison with transdermal route. *Maturitas* 2004;48:85–96.

Ettinger B, Ensrud KE, Wallace R, *et al*. Effects of ultralow-dose transdermal estradiol on bone mineral density: a randomized clinical trial. *Obstet Gynecol* 2004;**104**:443–51.

Grady D, Ettinger B, Tosteson AN, *et al*. Predictors of difficulty when discontinuing postmenopausal hormone therapy. *Obstet Gynecol* 2003;**102**:1233–9.

Graser T, Muller A, Mellinger U, *et al*. Continuous-combined treatment of the menopause with combinations of oestradiol valerate and dienogest – a dose-ranging study. *Maturitas* 2000;**35**:253–61.

Hampton N, Rees MC, Barlow DH, *et al*. Levonorgestrel intra-uterine system (LNG IUS) with conjugated oral equine oestrogen: a successful regimen for hormonal replacement therapy in perimenopausal women. *Hum Reprod* 2005;**20**:2653–60.

Haskell SG. After the Women's Health Initiative: postmenopausal women's experiences with discontinuing estrogen replacement therapy. *J Womens Health* 2004;**13**:438–42.

Heikkinen JE, Vaheri RT, Ahomaki SM, *et al*. Optimizing continuous-combined hormone replacement therapy for postmenopausal women: a comparison of six different treatment regimens. *Am J Obstet Gynecol* 2000;**182**:560–7.

Heikkinen J, Vaheri R, Kainulainen P, Timonen U. Long-term continuous combined hormone replacement therapy in the prevention of postmenopausal bone loss: a comparison of high- and low-dose estrogen-progestin regimens. *Osteoporos Int* 2000;**11**:929–37.

Hope S. Myalgia after stopping hormone replacement therapy. *J Br Menopause Soc* 2004;**10**:126.

Marshall SF, Hardy RJ, Kuh D. Socioeconomic variation in hysterectomy up to age 52: national, population based, prospective cohort study. *BMJ* 2000;**320**:1579.

Monthly Index of Medical Specialities. London: Haymarket Medical, 2005.

Nelson HD. Commonly used types of postmenopausal estrogen for treatment of hot flashes: scientific review. *JAMA* 2004;**291**:1610–20.

Ockene JK, Barad DH, Cochrane BB, *et al*. Symptom experience after discontinuing use of estrogen plus progestin. *JAMA* 2005;**294**:183–93.

Prestwood KM, Kenny AM, Kleppinger A, Kulldorff M. Ultralow-dose micronized 17beta-estradiol and bone density and bone metabolism in older women: a randomized controlled trial. *JAMA* 2003;**290**:1042–8.

Schurmann R, Holler T, Benda N. Estradiol and drospirenone for climacteric symptoms in postmenopausal women: a double-blind, randomized, placebo-controlled study of the safety and efficacy of three dose regimens. *Climacteric* 2004;**7**:189–96.

Shifren JL, Braunstein GD, Simon JA, *et al*. Transdermal testosterone treatment in women with impaired sexual function after oophorectomy. *N Engl J Med* 2000;**343**:682–8

Simunic V, Banovic I, Ciglar S, *et al*. Local estrogen treatment in patients with urogenital symptoms. *Int J Gynaecol Obstet* 2003;**82**:187–97.

Sitruk-Ware R. Pharmacological profile of progestins. *Maturitas* 2004;**47**:277–83.

Slater CC, Hodis HN, Mack WJ, *et al*. Markedly elevated levels of estrone sulfate after long-term oral, but not transdermal, administration of estradiol in postmenopausal women. *Menopause* 2001;**8**:200–3.

Sturdee DW, Rantala ML, Colau JC, *et al.* The acceptability of a small intrauterine progestogen-releasing system for continuous combined hormone therapy in early postmenopausal women. *Climacteric* 2004;7:404–11.

Suckling J, Lethaby A, Kennedy R. Local oestrogen for vaginal atrophy in postmenopausal women. *Cochrane Database Syst Rev* 2003;(4):CD001500.

Thakar R, Ayers S, Clarkson P, *et al.* Outcomes after total versus subtotal abdominal hysterectomy. *N Engl J Med* 2002;**347**:1318–25.

7 Benefits, risks and controversies regarding HRT

Designs of clinical trials
Women's Health Initiative and Million Women Studies
Benefits of HRT
Risks of HRT
Uncertainties
Further reading

Publication of the results of the Women's Health Initiative (WHI) and Million Women Study (MWS) since 2002 have led to considerable uncertainties about the role of hormone replacement therapy (HRT) among health professionals and women. This chapter will discuss types of study design, with special reference to the WHI and MWS.

Designs of clinical trials

Primary and secondary prevention trials

Primary prevention trials are those undertaken in healthy people, whereas secondary prevention trials involve participants with established medical conditions, such as cardiovascular disease and osteoporosis. It is important to distinguish between these two types of trials, as the responses may differ. For example, in women with cardiovascular disease, an endothelium with established atherosclerotic plaques is likely to respond differently from one without such plaques.

Randomized trials and cohort and case–control studies

Randomized trials
Randomized controlled trials (RCTs) are considered the best method for providing evidence on efficacy of an intervention. A perfectly randomized method to allocate participants to the study groups does not, however, protect an RCT from selection bias. Participants may not be typical of the whole population. In addition, differences may still exist between the groups studied – for example, in the number of smokers or types of drugs taken – and these can influence outcome. Randomized controlled trials, even if perfectly

designed, can tell us which treatment is better, but they cannot tell us for whom it is better. How and whether or not to generalize the results of a single trial to an individual patient is one of the most complex issues in healthcare. The findings that relate to a single drug treatment in a particular population thus cannot necessarily be extrapolated to all people. For example, the results of the WHI studies of HRT undertaken in women older than 50 years cannot be applied to women with a premature menopause.

In addition, RCTs tend to be short-term trials, and some interventions may take several years to have an effect. Also the behaviour of volunteer patients in trials may differ from those treated among the general public. Some of these problems can be overcome by cohort studies.

Cohort studies

Cohort studies can be thought of as natural experiments in which outcomes are measured in the real world rather than in experimental settings. They can evaluate large groups of diverse people, follow them for long periods and provide information on a range of outcomes, including rare adverse events. The promise of cohort studies as a useful source of evidence needs to be balanced, however, against concerns about the validity of that evidence. Cohort studies are similar to RCTs in that they compare outcomes in groups that did and did not receive an intervention. The main difference is that allocation of individuals is not by chance, so cohort studies are vulnerable to selection bias, which leads to criticism of the 'healthy user' effect, in which people with innately lower risks of an endpoint (such as myocardial infarction) as a result of good dietary and exercise habits may preferentially take the intervention under study – which then falsely gains credit for a favourable outcome. In cohort studies, therefore, factors that determine whether or not a person receives the intervention could result in the groups differing in factors related to the outcome – because people are selected preferentially to receive one treatment or because of choices they made. These baseline differences in prognosis could confound assessment of the effect of the intervention.

Case–control studies

In a case–control study, patients with a particular disease or condition (cases) are identified and 'matched' with controls (patients with some other disease, the general population, neighbours or relatives). Data are then collected (for example, by examining these people's medical records or asking them to recall their own history) about past exposure to a possible causal agent for the disease. Just as in cohort studies, case–control studies generally are concerned with the aetiology of a disease rather than its treatment. They lie lower down the hierarchy of evidence, but this design is usually the only practical option when studying rare conditions.

All observational studies, be they case–control or cohort in design, cannot prove causality – only association.

Explaining risk

Relative risk, absolute risk, attributable risk

Patients, the media and health professionals often confuse the terms 'relative risk', 'absolute risk' and 'attributable risk' (Box 7.1). An understanding of the precise definitions of these terms is important in order to judge the actual magnitude of risks involved. Epidemiological data that examine the risk of a disease often report 'relative risk' statistics to determine statistical significance. In other words, they report the risks run by a patient on a treatment relative to the risks run by a patient taking no treatment. This method provides substantial statistical power to detect effects of these agents, which might be quite small in magnitude. However it does not take into account the actual frequency of the condition in the untreated group. For example, a relative risk of 2 – often reported in the press as 'a doubling of risk' – could describe something that increases the risk of a disease from one in a million to two in a million or something that increases the risk of a disease from four people in 10 to eight people in 10. Thus 'absolute risk' and 'attributable risk' which take into account the frequency of the condition are better methods of presenting the data.

Hazard ratio and odds ratio

Risk also can be expressed as hazard and odds ratios. Hazard ratios (HR) broadly are equivalent to relative risk (RR) and are useful when the risk is not constant with respect to time. They use information collected at different times and were used in the publications from the WHI studies. The term is typically used in the context of survival over time. If the HR is 0.5, the RR of dying in one group is half the risk of dying in the other group.

Box 7.1

Relative risk, absolute risk and attributable risk

Relative risk is defined as the rate of disease among the treated group divided by the rate of the disease among the untreated group

Absolute risk is determined by multiplying the usual rate of the condition in the untreated group by the relative risk

Attributable risk is an absolute measure of the excess risk attributed to treatment. It is calculated as the difference in risk of a particular condition between those who are treated and those who are not

The odds ratio (OR) is the odds of an event happening in the treated group expressed as a proportion of the odds of an event happening in the untreated group. When events are rare, the OR is analogous to the RR, but as event rates increase, the OR and RR diverge.

Women's Health Initiative and Million Women Studies

Women's Health Initiative

The WHI is a large and complex clinical series of investigations of strategies for the prevention and control of some of the most common causes of morbidity and mortality among postmenopausal women, including cancer, cardiovascular disease and osteoporotic fractures. It was initiated in 1992, with a planned completion date of 2007. Postmenopausal women ranging in age from 50 to 79 years were enrolled at one of 40 clinical centres in the US into a clinical trial (CT) or observational study (OS). The CT was designed to allow randomized controlled evaluation of three distinct interventions (Box 7.2).

In the CT, the mean age of the women was 63 years.

The cohort of the OS comprised clinical trial screenees who were ineligible or unwilling to participate in the CT. The major clinical outcomes of interest in the OS are coronary heart disease (CHD), stroke, breast cancer, colorectal cancer, osteoporotic fractures, diabetes and total mortality.

Box 7.2

Interventions evaluated by Women's Health Initiative Clinical trial

- HRT (unopposed and combined) – hypothesized to reduce the risk of coronary heart disease (CHD) and other cardiovascular diseases and, secondarily, to reduce the risk of hip and other fractures, with increased risk of breast cancer being studied as a possible adverse outcome
- Low-fat eating pattern – hypothesized to prevent breast cancer and colorectal cancer and, secondarily, to prevent CHD
- Supplementation with calcium and vitamin D – hypothesized to prevent hip fractures and, secondarily, to prevent other fractures and colorectal cancer

---

Million Women Study

The MWS is an observational study that has evaluated the risk of breast cancer with respect to differences in HRT regimen and routes of administration (with the exception of vaginal preparations). Women invited to attend the NHS Breast Screening Programme (NHSBSP) were sent a self-administered questionnaire that asked them to document details about personal medical history and lifestyle factors, including the use of HRT. The study data were recorded from these questionnaires (which were returned before initial mammography), and women were followed to determine the incidence of cancer and death. A total of 1,084,110 women were recruited between 1996 and 2001; about half had ever used HRT. The average duration of follow up was 2.6 years. Several publications have questioned its design, analysis and conclusions, and a selection of comments is given below.

- The study reported a lower risk of breast cancer for perimenopausal and postmenopausal women than premenopausal women, despite the well-established fact that the risk of breast cancer increases with age.

- Many differences were present when women who used and did not use HRT were compared, and this required multiple adjustments.

- Use or non-use of HRT was established only at study entry and changes were not recorded during follow up. Lack of prospective follow up of exposure to HRT means that uncertainty exists as to whether women switched preparations or started or stopped HRT during the study's follow-up period.

- Validation of the questionnaire data was based on information obtained from only 570 women. Curiously, although the risk of endometrial cancer with unopposed oestrogen is well established, 14,024 non-hysterectomized women were documented as having taken HRT that contained oestrogen alone.

- Mortality from breast cancer was assessed after an average of 4.1 years of follow up and on the basis of a total of 517 deaths; however, breast cancer was diagnosed very rapidly, after a mean of 1.2 years, and deaths occurred swiftly (within an average of 1.7 years). This can be attributed to an underestimation of the total duration of exposure to HRT, as the risks presented were estimated on the basis of the use of HRT at recruitment. The study investigators did not adjust the total duration of use to account for the likely continued use of HRT in the period between recruitment and diagnosis of cancer (that is, a mean of 1.2 years). Current users and past users of HRT were compared with never users, and, although the risk of mortality was increased, it was not significant (RR 1.22, 95% confidence interval 1.00 to 1.48). This finding was highlighted because it differed from consistent reports in the literature over a decade that women who take hormones have better survival rates. The MWS calculated the risk of mortality by dividing deaths from breast cancer by the total number of women who used HRT or those who did not. If the risk is recalculated by dividing deaths from breast cancer by the total number of cases of breast cancer in women who did and did not use HRT, the results agree with the literature – the risk of mortality was reduced by about 27% in the women who took hormones.

- The higher estimates of risk reported compared with those from the randomized WHI study – especially the oestrogen-alone arm, which found a reduced risk – probably reflects the observational nature of the MWS and suggests that the latter study probably grossly overestimated the risk of breast cancer.

- The data provided are probably representative of about 25% of all women aged 50–64 years in the UK (on the basis of uptake for the first prevalent NHSBSP round of 75%, completion of the MWS' questionnaire by 50% of attendees and the number of screening centres in the UK that participated in the study (66/94)). Differences between women who did and did not attend the NHSBSP and between attendees who agreed – or declined – to participate in the study cannot easily be controlled for.

Benefits of HRT

Vasomotor symptoms

Good evidence from randomized placebo-controlled studies, including WHI, shows that oestrogen is effective in treating hot flushes and that improvement is usually noted within four weeks. Maximum therapeutic response to any particular formulation is usually achieved by three months, at which point progress should be reviewed critically. Treatment should be continued for at least one year; otherwise, symptoms often recur. Relief of vasomotor symptoms is the most common indication for a prescription of HRT and is often used for less than five years.

Urogenital symptoms and sexuality

Symptoms such as vaginal dryness, soreness, superficial dyspareunia and urinary frequency and urgency respond well to oestrogens, which may be given topically or systemically. Recurrent urinary tract infections may be prevented by oestrogen replacement, but the appropriate dose and duration of therapy have yet to be identified. Improvement may take several months. Long-term treatment is often needed, as symptoms can recur on cessation of treatment. Urinary incontinence, however, is not improved by systemic therapy. Sexuality may be improved with oestrogen alone, but it may also need the addition of testosterone – by implant only at present – especially in young oophorectomized women (see Chapter 6).

Osteoporosis

Evidence from randomized controlled trials (including WHI) shows that HRT reduces the risk of spine and hip fractures, as well as other osteoporotic fractures. Most epidemiological studies suggest that continuous and lifelong use is required for HRT to be an effective method of preventing fracture. Regulatory authorities (December 2003) have advised that HRT should not be used as a first-line treatment for osteoporosis prevention, as the risks outweigh the benefits. This may be true for a population with no increased risk of osteoporosis (as in WHI), but the risk–benefit ratio changes favourably when a population with increased risk of osteoporosis is targeted. Although alternatives to HRT are available for the prevention and treatment of osteoporosis in elderly women, oestrogen may remain the best option, particularly in women who are younger or symptomatic, or both. The 'standard' doses of oestrogen said to be bone protective were oestradiol 1–2 mg, conjugated equine oestrogens 0.625 mg and transdermal 25–50 µg patch. It is now evident, however, that half of these doses are protective. Some women have no bone response to HRT, despite good compliance with therapy. Current smokers and women with low body weight seem to be at increased risk of poor bone response to HRT. Although tibolone conserves bone mass, data on fractures are awaited and will be required before this agent could be licensed for this purpose.

Few data are available on the efficacy of alternatives such as bisphosphonates in perimenopausal or early postmenopausal women. Currently, HRT is significantly cheaper to prescribe than alternative therapies, such as bisphosphonates, strontium ranelate and parathyroid hormone.

Colorectal cancer

Data from the oestrogen–progestogen arm, but not the oestrogen-alone arm, of the WHI study were consistent with data from case–control and cohort studies that showed that HRT reduces the risk of colorectal cancer by about one-third. Little is known, however, about the risk of colorectal cancer when treatment is stopped. No information is available about HRT in high-risk populations, and current data do not allow prevention of colonic cancer as a recommendation for HRT.

Risks of HRT

Breast cancer

Breast cancer is a common condition, with a lifetime risk (up to age 85 years) in the UK of one in nine (Table 7.1). The pattern of incidence of breast cancer supports a link with endogenous sex hormones, as rates increase steeply before the menopause and, although they continue to rise after ovarian function has ceased, they do so less rapidly. Age is the most important risk factor; however, as most breast cancers (80%) are diagnosed in people older than 50 years. In the UK, the overall risk of breast cancer in 2000 was 114 per

100,000 female population; currently, it is the most common female malignancy. Despite the fact that most women diagnosed with breast cancer are alive five years after diagnosis and treatment, women understandably are concerned about any factors that may increase their risk of breast cancer and this is the most common reason given for not wanting to use HRT in the long term. Since 1989, mortality from breast cancer in the UK has decreased significantly (age standardized death rates have reduced by 29%: from 42 per 100,000 women in 1989 to 29 per 100,000 women in 2003). This decrease has been attributed to the more widespread use of adjuvant treatment for breast cancer and the introduction of mammographic screening programmes to detect breast cancer.

Overall, HRT seems to confer a similar degree of risk to that associated with late natural menopause. For every year that the menopause is delayed, the risk of breast cancer increases by 2.8%. With HRT, the risk has been estimated to increase by 2.3% per year. Epidemiological and randomized studies suggest that the risk of developing breast cancer with HRT is dependent on duration of treatment, but that this effect is not sustained once HRT is stopped, when

Table 7.1

Breast cancer risk. Adapted from American Cancer Society (2004)

Relative risk (RR)	Risk factor
High risk (RR >4)	• Certain inherited genetic mutations, eg BRCA1 or BRCA2 • Personal history of breast cancer • Biopsy confirmed atypical hyperplasia* • High dose radiation to chest (mantle radiotherapy for Hodgkin's at age <35 years)
Moderate risk (RR 2–4)	• Family history (see Chapter 5)
Low increased risk (RR 1.1–2)	• Benign breast disease without evidence of epithelial atypia • Recent and long-term use of hormone replacement therapy • Late age at first full term pregnancy (>30 years) • Early menarche (<12 years) • Late menopause (>55 years) • Nulliparity • Alcohol consumption • Postmenopausal obesity • High socioeconomic status

*This is a risk marker, ie risk of subsequent breast cancer affects both breasts (Chapter 12)

the risk after five years is no greater than that in women who have never been exposed to HRT. All risk estimates are based on commencement of HRT at the age of 50 years, as such an effect is not seen in women who start HRT early for a premature menopause, which indicates that the duration of lifetime exposure to female sex hormones (for example, oestrogen and progestogen) is relevant. The risk of breast cancer with HRT is dependent on the regimen prescribed. Risk seems to be greatest with combined oestrogen–progestogen replacement and less so with unopposed oestrogen. Combined HRT probably accounts for an extra three breast cancers per 1000 women who start it at the age of 50 years and use it for five years. The increased risk of breast cancer with combined therapy compared with oestrogen treatment has to be balanced against the reduction in risk of endometrial cancer provided by combined therapy. The increased risk of breast cancer with longer term exposure seems to be limited in most studies to lean women (that is, those with a BMI <25 kg/m^2). It also must be remembered that the increase in risk of breast cancer found in nulliparous women, those with a high BMI, those who delay their first birth and those who have a family history of breast cancer may be higher than that conferred by HRT.

The Women's Health Initiative found:

- The risk of breast cancer in the oestrogen-alone group (that is, the group of women who used conjugated equine oestrogen only) was 23% lower than in the placebo group. In absolute terms, this represents four fewer cases of breast cancer per 1000 women on an intention to treat analysis for five years at 50–59 years, five fewer at 60–69 years and one less case at 70–79 years.
- In the combined HRT group, evidence of an effect of duration was seen. An increase in risk began to emerge three years after randomization but only in women with a history of using HRT before study entry. In absolute terms, the excess or attributable risk in the WHI study with combined therapy was three cases of breast cancer per 1000 women on an intention to treat analysis of five years at age 50–59 years, four at 60–69 years and seven at 70–79 years (Table 7.2).

The Million Women Study found:

- an increased risk of breast cancer with all HRT regimens (that is, unopposed oestrogen, combined HRT, and tibolone)
- the greatest degree of risk with combined HRT; this was not influenced by route of administration
- the pattern of progestogen administration (cyclical or continuous) or a change in the oestrogen or progestogen did not seem to affect risk.

Table 7.2

Breast cancer risk per 1000 women from intention-to-treat analysis of five years of data from the Women's Health Initiative studies

| Age range (years) | Risk of breast cancer per 1000 women | | | | |
| | Oestrogen only | | Continuous combined hormone replacement therapy | | |
	Hazard ratio (95% confidence interval)	Difference	Hazard ratio (95% confidence interval)	Difference
50–59	0.72 (0.43 to 1.21)	−4 (−7 to +3)	1.20 (0.80 to 1.82)	+3 (−3 to +11)
60–69	0.72 (0.49 to 1.07)	−5 (−9 to +1)	1.22 (0.90 to 1.66)	+4 (−2 to +12)
70–79	0.94 (0.56 to 1.60)	−1 (−9 to +12)	1.34 (0.88 to 2.04)	+7 (−2 to +21)
All	0.77 (0.59 to 1.01)	−4 (−7 to 0)	1.24 (1.01 to 1.54)	+4 (0 to +9)

Mortality from breast cancer

Mortality from breast cancer is the most important outcome (Table 7.3). No randomized trial, including WHI, is ever likely to be large enough to evaluate this endpoint reliably. Advice about the effect of HRT on survival in women with breast cancer has to be drawn from observational studies or predictions of outcome made on the basis of the biological characteristics of tumours, or both. Overall, observational studies suggest that use of HRT has no significant effect on survival compared with non-use of HRT and indeed may improve it. The MWS reported an increased mortality in current users of HRT, but this was of borderline significance and, in the absence of information about tumour pathology, stage and treatment, any definitive conclusions are difficult to draw. The WHI study reported that cancers associated with combined HRT were significantly larger and more likely to be node positive than cancers associated with placebo. The mean difference in tumour size, however, was only 2 mm, and the number of events from which the data on lymph node was estimated was small and confidence intervals wide. On the basis of data from the WHI study, the estimated survival difference at 10 years is very small (1.5%).

Table 7.3

Combined hormone replacement therapy and mortality from breast cancer for 5 years use per 1000 women based on the WHI study

Age range (years)	Continuous combined hormone replacement therapy	
	Hazard ratio	Absolute difference in number of deaths
50–59	1.25	+1.4
60–69	1.27	+1.5
70–79	1.39	+2.2
All	1.32	+1.8

In discussion with women on this key issue, it is important to stick to absolute values and if possible have charts available showing the background rate of breast cancer and the extra cases anticipated with combined HRT. It is also important to note that the oestrogen-alone arm of WHI found no excess of breast cancer cases in the oestrogen-treated women.

Endometrial cancer

The link between unopposed oestrogen replacement therapy and endometrial cancer was established more than 20 years ago. The relative risk (RR) is 2.3, increases with prolonged duration of use (RR 9.5 for ≥10 years)

and remains increased for five or more years after discontinuation of unopposed oestrogen therapy (RR 2.3). The increased risk of endometrial cancer in women who use HRT has to be compared with that found in obese and diabetic women, where it is higher.

Furthermore, oral, but not vaginal, treatment with low-potency oestrogen formulations (such as oestriol) increases the relative risk of endometrial neoplasia (Table 7.4). The excess relative risk with low-potency oestrogen is lost rapidly after treatment stops.

Although one study in 417 women over two years shows that very low-dose oestrogen does not seem to stimulate the endometrium, this needs to be confirmed with larger numbers and over a longer period of time. It would be premature, therefore, to recommend this regimen in non-hysterectomized women.

The addition of progestogen has been advocated for many years, with the intention of reducing the risk of hyperplasia and carcinoma. Most studies have shown that this excess risk is not eliminated completely with the addition of monthly sequential progestogen, especially when it is continued for more than five years. This also has been found with long-cycle HRT. No increased risk of endometrial cancer has been found with continuous combined regimens. Debate surrounds the relative merits of different progestogens; however, studies have not examined equivalent doses. Although laboratory studies and clinical trials show that tibolone induces endometrial atrophy, the MWS and a case–control study from the UK General Practice Research Database have shown an increased risk of endometrial cancer. Further studies are awaited.

Table 7.4

Endometrial cancer risk and hormone replacement therapy after five or more years of use. Data derived from Weiderpass (1999a and 1999b)

Type of hormone replacement therapy	Odds ratio (95% confidence interval)
Oestradiol alone	6.2 (3.1 to 12.6)
Conjugated oestrogens	6.6 (3.6 to 12.0)
Cyclic use of progestogens plus oestrogen – that is, fewer than 16 days per cycle (most commonly 10 days)	2.9 (1.8 to 4.6)
Continuous progestogen use along with oestrogens	0.2 (0.1 to 0.8)
Oral oestriol 1–2 mg daily	3.0 (2.0 to 4.4)
Low potency vaginal oestrogens	1.2 (0.8 to 1.9)

Venous thromboembolism

Until 1996, HRT, unlike the combined oral contraceptive pill, was not suspected to increase the risk of venous thromboembolism (VTE). Although HRT reduces fibrinogen and increases the natural anticoagulant protein C, it also decreases the natural anticoagulants antithrombin and protein S and increases factors VII and VIII and von Willebrand factor. We now know that the overall effect is to increase the propensity to VTE. The best evidence comes from the Heart and Estrogen/progestin Replacement Study (HERS) and WHI randomized prospective studies. For combined therapy, the OR was 2.7 (1.4 to 5.0) in HERS and 2.1 (1.6 to 2.7) in WHI. These OR are slightly lower than those for the second-generation combined oral contraceptives. The highest risk occurs in the first year of use. The absolute risk is small, however, as VTE occurs in 1.7 per 1000 in women older than 50 years who are not taking HRT and mortality is low (1–2%). Advancing age, obesity and an underlying thrombophilia, such as Factor V Leiden, significantly increase risk. For example, in the placebo arm of the WHI, the number of cases of VTE per 1000 women per year was 0.8 at 50–59 years, 1.9 at 60–69 years and 2.7 at 70–79 years.

In women who have taken HRT after VTE, data from randomized trials show an increased risk of recurrence in the first year that the hormone is used. Limited data suggest that transdermal HRT seems to be associated with a lower risk than oral therapy.

No large clinical trials are available yet regarding the effects of tibolone on VTE. Some experimental data suggest that tibolone may not have the same prothrombotic effects as oestrogen-based HRT. Further research is required, however, before definite conclusions can be reached about the risk of VTE with tibolone.

Gallbladder disease

The WHI confirmed the observation published by HERS in 1998 that HRT increases the risk of gallbladder disease. Gallbladder disease increases with age and obesity, and, as a confounder, women who use HRT may have a silent pre-existing disease.

Uncertainties

Cardiovascular disease (coronary heart disease and stroke)

Until the late 1990s, oestrogen was thought to protect against cardiovascular disease. Many cohort studies have shown that HRT results in a reduction in the incidence of CHD of around 40–50%. The effect does not seem to be lost when progestogen is added. Concerns that the apparent reduction of CHD with HRT reflected a healthy user bias have been addressed by large studies, in which cases and controls were matched for lifestyle factors and major risk factors. Oestrogen replacement has also been found to be beneficial in postmenopausal women with established CHD: a 50–80% reduction in the incidence of CHD and an increase in survival have been reported. The greatest benefit in terms of survival was seen in women with the most severe coronary artery disease. Results from randomized controlled trials for primary or secondary prevention, however, have not confirmed the results of these observational studies. Thus the role of HRT in primary or secondary prevention is now uncertain, and it should not be used primarily for this indication at this time.

Coronary heart disease

Primary prevention
Women who took combined HRT in the WHI study showed an early, albeit transient, increase in coronary events. The attributable risk at 50–59 years was five cases of non-fatal myocardial infarction and death due to CHD per 10,000 women per year, at 60–69 years was one, and at 70–79 years was 23. The oestrogen-alone arm of WHI showed neither risk nor benefit, although there was a tendency for a reduction in events in the younger women. The reduced attributable risk was 10 cases at 50–59 years and five at 60–69 years, with an excess risk of four cases in those aged 70–79 years.

The timing, dose and possibly type of HRT, however, may be critical in determining cardiovascular effects, as found in the WHI and prospective cohort Nurses' Health Study. Women in the WHI study who started combined HRT within 10 years of the menopause had a lower risk of CHD than women who started later (Figure 7.1).

In WHI, the same HRT regimen was used in all non-hysterectomized women regardless of age: conjugated equine oestrogens 0.625 mg combined with medroxyprogesterone acetate 2.5 mg. A possible explanation for early cardiovascular harm associated with HRT is an increase in thrombogenesis or abnormal cardiovascular remodelling. Both of these effects are dose dependent. Thus, although oestrogen has the potential to cause vascular benefit (as shown in observational and animal studies), high doses have the potential to cause vascular harm. The starting dose, type of hormone and route of administration may thus be critical in determining the effect on CHD. The results of the oestrogen-alone arm of WHI are consistent with this hypothesis: reduced risk was found in women aged 50–69 years and increased risk in older women. The dose of oestrogen used in WHI was thus inappropriately high for older women. The differences between the findings of randomized trials and observational studies may result from the fact that

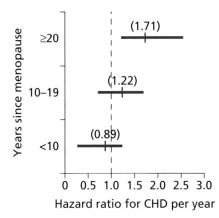

Figure 7.1 Influence of time since menopause on the effect of hormone replacement therapy on coronary heart disease. Adapted from Manson *et al.* (2003)

the latter mainly include women who start HRT around the time of the menopause, with doses appropriate to their age.

Secondary prevention

Although angiographic and cohort studies, such as the Nurses' Health Study, suggested a role of oestrogen in the secondary prevention of CHD, this has not been confirmed in randomized controlled trials (Table 7.5).

Stroke

A substantial body of observational data are available on HRT and stroke. Interpretation is complicated, however, by the differences in study design, failure to differentiate between ischaemic and haemorrhagic stroke and the status of HRT use (current users versus ever users). The observational Nurses' Health Study showed no increase in the incidence of stroke except when high-dose oestrogen was used. Similarly, the HERS investigators reported no increase in stroke in their randomized controlled trial.

Both active arms of WHI found an increase in ischaemic but not haemorrhagic stroke. The excess absolute risk for the combined HRT arm was four cases of stroke per 10,000 women per year at 50–59 years, nine at 60–69 years and 13 at 70–79 years. The excess absolute risk for the oestrogen-alone arm was 0 cases of stroke per 10,000 women per year at 50–59 years, 19 at 60–69 years and 14 at 70–79 years.

In women who have already experienced a previous ischaemic stroke, oestrogen replacement does not reduce mortality or recurrence, as evidenced by data from randomized controlled trials.

Table 7.5

Randomized controlled trials of hormone replacement therapy as secondary prevention for coronary heart disease. CEE, conjugated equine oestrogens. MPA, medroxyprogesterone acetate.

Study	Hormone replacement therapy	Route of administration	Relative risk (95% confidence interval) of acute myocardial infarction	Sample size
HERS (Hulley, 1998)	CEE/MPA	Oral	0.99 (0.8 to 1.22)	2769
PHASE (Clarke, 2002)	17β-oestradiol	Transdermal	1.29 (0.84 to 1.95)	255
WEST (Viscoli, 2001)	17β-oestradiol	Oral	1.1 (0.6 to 1.9)	664
ESPRIT (Cherry, 2002)	Oestradiol valerate	Oral	0.99 (0.7 to 1.41)	1017

Dementia and cognition

Although oestrogen may delay or reduce the risk of Alzheimer's disease, it does not seem to improve established disease. Whether a critical age or duration of treatment exists for oestrogen to have an effect in prevention is unclear. However, a window of opportunity may be present in the early postmenopause, when the pathological processes that lead to Alzheimer's disease (and cardiovascular disease) are being initiated and when HRT may have a preventive effect. The WHI found a two-fold increased risk of dementia in women with oestrogen and progestogen and oestrogen alone; however, this increased risk was only significant in the group of women older than 75 years. Similarly, WHI found deterioration in cognitive function in women older than 65 years, especially in those with lower cognitive function at the start of treatment. Why these results are the opposite of earlier findings from observational studies and animal models is unclear. More evidence is needed, especially from younger postmenopausal women who take appropriate doses and different regimens, before definitive advice can be given in relation to dementia and cognition.

Ovarian cancer

Most data pertain to replacement with oestrogen alone, with increasing risk in the very long term (>10 years). With continuous combined therapy, however, this increase does not seem apparent. This issue is unresolved and requires further examination and currently insufficient evidence is available to recommend alterations in HRT prescribing practice.

Quality of life

Although some studies have shown improvement in both symptomatic and asymptomatic women, others have not. This area is difficult to evaluate because of the different measures used, varying levels of menopausal symptoms, a large placebo effect and extrinsic factors that may alter women's responses.

Further reading

General

Banks E, Beral V, Cameron R, *et al.* Agreement between general practice prescription data and self-reported use of hormone replacement therapy and treatment for various illnesses. *J Epidemiol Biostat* 2001;6:357–63.

Beral V, Bull D, Reeves G; Million Women Study Collaborators. Endometrial cancer and hormone-replacement therapy in the Million Women Study. *Lancet* 2005;365:1543–51.

Garton M. Breast cancer and hormone-replacement therapy: the Million Women Study. *Lancet* 2003;**362**:1328–31

Greenhalgh T. How to read a paper: assessing the methodological quality of published papers. *BMJ* 1997;**315**:305–8

Jadad AR. *Randomised Controlled Trials: A User's Guide.* London: BMJ Books, 1998.

Million Women Study Collaborators. Breast cancer and hormone-replacement therapy in the Million Women Study. *Lancet* 2003;**362**:419–27.

NHS Breast Screening Review 2004, www.cancerscreening.nhs.uk (last accessed 29 September 2005)

Rochon PA, Gurwitz JH, Sykora K, *et al.* Reader's guide to critical appraisal of cohort studies: 1. Role and design. *BMJ* 2005;**330**:895–7.

Santen RJ. Risk of breast cancer with progestins: critical assessment of current data. *Steroids* 2003;**68**:953–64.

Speroff L. A clinician's review of the WHI-related literature. *Int J Fertil Womens Med* 2004;**49**:252–67.

The Million Women Study Collaborators. The Million Women Study: design and characteristics of the study population. *Breast Cancer Res* 1999;**1**:73–80

The Women's Health Initiative Study Group. Design of the Women's Health Initiative clinical trial and observational study. *Control Clin Trials* 1998;**19**:61–109.

The Women's Health Initiative Steering Committee. Effects of conjugated equine estrogen in postmenopausal women with hysterectomy: the Women's Health Initiative randomized controlled trial. *JAMA* 2004;**291**:1701–12.

Whitehead M, Farmer R. The Million Women Study: a critique. *Endocrine* 2004;**24**:187–93.

Writing Group for the Women's Health Initiative Investigators. Risks and benefits of estrogen plus progestin in healthy postmenopausal women: principal results from the Women's Health Initiative randomized controlled trial. *JAMA* 2002;**288**:321–33.

Vasomotor symptoms

Barnabei VM, Cochrane BB, Aragaki AK, *et al.* Menopausal symptoms and treatment-related effects of estrogen and progestin in the Women's Health Initiative. *Obstet Gynecol* 2005;**105**:1063–73.

Maclennan A, Broadbent J, Lester S, Moore V. Oral oestrogen and combined oestrogen/progestogen therapy versus placebo for hot flushes. *Cochrane Database Syst Rev* 2004;(**4**):CD002978.

Nelson HD. Commonly used types of postmenopausal estrogen for treatment of hot flashes: scientific review. *JAMA* 2004;**291**:1610–20.

Urogenital symptoms and sexuality

Brown JS, Vittinghoff E, Kanaya AM, *et al.* Heart and Estrogen/Progestin Replacement Study Research Group. Urinary tract infections in postmenopausal women: effect of hormone therapy and risk factors. *Obstet Gynecol* 2001;**98**:1045–52.

Cardozo L, Bachmann G, McClish D, *et al.* Meta-analysis of estrogen therapy in the management of urogenital atrophy in postmenopausal women: second report of the Hormones and Urogenital Therapy Committee. *Obstet Gynecol* 1998;**92**:722–7.

Floter A, Nathorst-Boos J, Carlstrom K, von Schoultz B. Addition of testosterone to estrogen replacement therapy in oophorectomized women: effects on sexuality and well-being. *Climacteric* 2002;**5**:357–65.

Grady D, Brown JS, Vittinghoff E, *et al.*; HERS Research Group. Postmenopausal hormones and incontinence: the Heart and Estrogen/Progestin Replacement Study. *Obstet Gynecol* 2001;**97**:116–20.

Hendrix SL, Cochrane BB, Nygaard IE, *et al.* Effects of estrogen with and without progestin on urinary incontinence. *JAMA* 2005;**293**:935–48.

Osteoporosis

Bagger YZ, Tanko LB, Alexandersen P, *et al.* Two to three years of hormone replacement treatment in healthy women have long-term preventive effects on bone mass and osteoporotic fractures: the PERF study. *Bone* 2004;**34**:728–35.

Cauley JA, Robbins J, Chen Z, *et al.* Effects of estrogen plus progestin on risk of fracture and bone mineral density: the Women's Health Initiative randomized trial. *JAMA* 2003;**290**:1729–38.

Ettinger B, Ensrud KE, Wallace R, *et al.* Effects of ultralow-dose transdermal estradiol on bone mineral density: a randomized clinical trial. *Obstet Gynecol* 2004; **104**:443–51.

Francis RM. Non-response to osteoporosis treatment. *J Br Menopause Soc* 2004; **10**:76–80.

Heikkinen J, Vaheri R, Kainulainen P, Timonen U. Long-term continuous combined hormone replacement therapy in the prevention of postmenopausal bone loss: a comparison of high- and low-dose estrogen-progestin regimens. *Osteoporos Int* 2000;**11**:929–37.

Hundrup YA, Hoidrup S, Ekholm O, *et al.* Risk of low-energy hip, wrist, and upper arm fractures among current and previous users of hormone replacement therapy: The Danish Nurse Cohort Study. *Eur J Epidemiol* 2004;**19**:1089–95.

Komulainen MH, Kroger H, Tuppurainen MT, *et al.* HRT and Vit D in prevention of non-vertebral fractures in postmenopausal women: a 5 year randomised trial. *Maturitas* 1998;**31**:45–54.

Lufkin EG, Wahner HW, O'Fallon WM, *et al.* Treatment of postmenopausal osteoporosis with transdermal estrogen. *Ann Intern Med* 1992;**117**:1–9.

Prestwood KM, Kenny AM, Kleppinger A, Kulldorff M. Ultralow-dose micronized 17beta-estradiol and bone density and bone metabolism in older women: a randomized controlled trial. *JAMA* 2003;**290**:1042–8.

Royal College of Physicians. *Osteoporosis: Clinical Guidelines for Prevention and Treatment. Update on Pharmacological Interventions and an Algorithm for Management.* London: Royal College of Physicians, 2000. http://www.rcplondon.ac.uk/ (last accessed 29 September 2005).

Torgerson DJ, Bell-Syer SE. Hormone replacement therapy and prevention of nonvertebral fractures: a meta-analysis of randomized trials. *JAMA* 2001; **285**:2891–7.

Colorectal cancer

Fernandez E, Franceschi S, La Vecchia C. Colorectal cancer and hormone replacement therapy: a review of epidemiological studies. *J Br Menopause Soc* 2000;6:8–14.

Herbert-Croteau N. A meta-analysis of hormone replacement therapy and colon cancer in women. *Cancer Epidemiol Biomarkers Prev* 1998;7:653–9.

The Women's Health Initiative Steering Committee. Effects of conjugated equine estrogen in postmenopausal women with hysterectomy: the Women's Health Initiative randomized controlled trial. *JAMA* 2004;**291**:1701–12.

Writing Group for the Women's Health Initiative Investigators. Risks and benefits of estrogen plus progestin in healthy postmenopausal women: principal results from the Women's Health Initiative randomized controlled trial. *JAMA* 2002; **288**:321–33.

Breast cancer

American Cancer Society. *Breast Cancer Facts and Figures, 2003–2004.* Atlanta, GA: American Cancer Society, 2004. Available at: http://www.cancer.org (last accessed 20 September 2005).

Bush TL, Whiteman M, Flaws JA. Hormone replacement therapy and breast cancer: a qualitative review. *Obstet Gynecol* 2001;**98**:498–508.

Chlebowski RT, Hendrix SL, Langer RD, *et al.* Influence of estrogen plus progestin on breast cancer and mammography in healthy postmenopausal women. The Women's Health Initiative randomized trial. *JAMA* 2003;**289**:3243–53.

Collaborative Group on Hormonal Factors in Breast Cancer 1997. Breast Cancer and HRT: collaborative reanalysis of data from 51 epidemiological studies of 52,705 women with breast cancer and 108,411 women without breast cancer. *Lancet* 1997;**350**:1047–59

La Vecchia C, Brinton LA, McTiernan A. Cancer risk in menopausal women. *Best Pract Res Clin Obstet Gynaecol* 2002;**16**:293–307.

Magnusson C, Baron JA, Correia N, *et al.* Breast-cancer risk following long-term oestrogen- and oestrogen-progestin-replacement therapy. *Int J Cancer* 1999; **81**:339–44.

Manjer J, Malina J, Berglund G, *et al.* Increased incidence of small and well-differentiated breast tumours in post-menopausal women following hormone-replacement therapy. *Int J Cancer* 2001;**92**:919–22

Million Women Study Collaborators. Breast cancer and hormone-replacement therapy in the Million Women Study. *Lancet* 2003;**362**:419–27.

Ross RK, Paganini-Hill A, Wan PC, Pike MC. Effect of hormone replacement therapy on breast cancer risk: estrogen versus estrogen plus progestin. *J Natl Cancer Inst* 2000;**92**:328–32

Santen RJ, Pinkerton J, McCartney C, Petroni GR. Risk of breast cancer with progestins in combination with estrogen as hormone replacement therapy. *J Clin Endocrinol Metab* 2001;**86**:16–23.

Schairer C, Lubin J, Troisi R, *et al.* Menopausal estrogen and estrogen-progestin replacement therapy and breast cancer risk. *JAMA* 2000;**283**:485–91.

The Women's Health Initiative Steering Committee. Effects of conjugated equine estrogen in postmenopausal women with hysterectomy: the Women's Health Initiative randomized controlled trial. *JAMA* 2004;**291**:1701–12.

Willis DB, Calle EE, Miracle-McMahill HL, Heath CW. Estrogen replacement therapy and risk of fatal breast cancer in a prospective cohort of postmenopausal women in the United States. *Cancer Causes Control* 1996;7:449–57

Endometrial cancer

Anderson GL, Judd HL, Kaunitz AM, *et al*; Women's Health Initiative Investigators. Effects of estrogen plus progestin on gynecologic cancers and associated diagnostic procedures: the Women's Health Initiative randomized trial. *JAMA* 2003; **290**:1739–48.

Beral V, Bull D, Reeves G; Million Women Study Collaborators. Endometrial cancer and hormone-replacement therapy in the Million Women Study. *Lancet* 2005;**365**:1543–51.

Beresford SA, Weiss NS, Voigt LF, *et al*. Risk of endometrial cancer in relation to use of oestrogen combined with cyclic progestogen therapy in post menopausal women. *Lancet* 1997;**349**:458–61

Brinton L, Hoover R. Estrogen replacement therapy and endometrial cancer: unresolved issues. *Obstet Gynecol* 1993;**81**:265–71.

Erkkola R, Kumento U, Lehmuskoski S, *et al*. No increased risk of endometrial hyperplasia with fixed long-cycle oestrogen-progestogen therapy after five years. *J Br Menopause Soc* 2004;**10**:9–13.

Grady D, Gebretsadik T, Kerlikowske K, *et al*. Hormone replacement therapy and endometrial cancer risk: a meta-analysis. *Obstet Gynecol* 1995;**85**:304–13.

Johnson SR, Ettinger B, Macer JL, *et al*. Uterine and vaginal effects of unopposed ultralow-dose transdermal estradiol. *Obstet Gynecol* 2005;**105**:779–87.

Lethaby A, Suckling J, Barlow D, *et al*. Hormone replacement therapy in postmenopausal women: endometrial hyperplasia and irregular bleeding. *Cochrane Database Syst Rev* 2004;(3):CD000402.

Pike MC, Peters RK, Cozen W, *et al*. Estrogen-progestin replacement therapy and endometrial cancer. *J Natl Cancer Inst* 1997;**89**:1110–16

Pukkala E, Tulenheimo-Silfvast A, Leminen A. Incidence of cancer among women using long versus monthly cycle hormonal replacement therapy, Finland 1994–1997. *Cancer Causes Control* 2001;**12**:111–15.

Reed SD, Voigt LF, Beresford SA, *et al*. Dose of progestin in postmenopausal-combined hormone therapy and risk of endometrial cancer. *Am J Obstet Gynecol* 2004; **191**:1146–51.

Sturdee DW, Ulrich LG, Barlow DH, *et al*. The endometrial response to sequential and continuous combined oestrogen-progestogen replacement therapy. *BJOG* 2000;**107**:1392–400.

de Vries CS, Bromley SE, Thomas H, Farmer RD. Tibolone and endometrial cancer: a cohort and nested case-control study in the UK. *Drug Saf* 2005;**28**:241–9.

Weiderpass E, Adami HO, Baron JA, *et al*. Risk of endometrial cancer following estrogen replacement with and without progestins. *J Natl Cancer Inst* 1999a;**91**:1131–7.

Weiderpass E, Baron JA, Adami HO, *et al.* Low-potency oestrogen and risk of endometrial cancer: a case-control study. *Lancet* 1999b;353:1824–8.

Weiderpass E, Persson I, Adami HO, *et al.* Body size in different periods of life, diabetes mellitus, hypertension, and risk of postmenopausal endometrial cancer (Sweden). *Cancer Causes Control* 2000;11:185–92.

Venous thromboembolism

Cushman M, Kuller LH, Prentice R, *et al*; Women's Health Initiative Investigators. Estrogen plus progestin and risk of venous thrombosis. *JAMA* 2004;292:1573–80.

Daly E, Vessey MP, Hawkins MM, *et al.* Risk of venous thromboembolism in users of hormone replacement therapy. *Lancet* 1996;348:977–80.

Douketis JD, Julian JA, Kearon C, *et al.* Does the type of hormone replacement therapy influence the risk of deep vein thrombosis? A prospective case-control study. *J Thromb Haemost* 2005;3:943–8.

Hoibraaten E, Qvigstad E, Arnesen H, *et al.* Increased risk of recurrent venous thromboembolism during hormone replacement therapy – results of the random-ized, double-blind, placebo-controlled estrogen in venous thromboembolism trial (EVTET). *Thromb Haemost* 2000;84:961–7.

Hulley S, Grady D, Bush T, *et al.* Randomized trial of estrogen plus progestin for secondary prevention of coronary heart disease in postmenopausal women. Heart and Estrogen/progestin Replacement Study (HERS) Research Group. *JAMA* 1998;280:605–13.

Jick H, Derby LE, Myers MW, *et al.* Risk of hospital admission for idiopathic venous thromboembolism among users of postmenopausal oestrogens. *Lancet* 1996;348:981–3.

Keeling DM. Hormone replacement therapy, thrombosis and thrombophilia. *J Br Menopause Soc* 2005;11:74–5.

Lowe G, Woodward M, Vessey M, *et al.* Thrombotic variables and risk of idiopathic venous thromboembolism in women aged 45–64 years. Relationships to hormone replacement therapy. *Thromb Haemost* 2000;83:530–5.

Royal College of Obstetricians and Gynaecologists. *Hormone Replacement Therapy and Venous Thromboembolism.* London: Royal College of Obstetricians and Gynaecologists, 2004.

Scarabin PY, Oger E, Plu-Bureau G, *et al.* Differential association of oral and transdermal oestrogen-replacement therapy with venous thromboembolism risk. *Lancet* 2003;362:428–32.

Varas-Lorenzo C, Garcia-Rodriguez LA, Cattaruzzi C, *et al.* Hormone replacement therapy and the risk of hospitalization for venous thromboembolism: a population-based study in southern Europe. *Am J Epidemiol* 1998;147:387–90.

Winkler UH, Altkemper R, Kwee B, *et al.* Effects of tibolone and continuous combined hormone replacement therapy on parameters in the clotting cascade: a multicenter, double-blind, randomized study. *Fertil Steril* 2000;74:10–19.

Gallbladder disease

Cirillo DJ, Wallace RB, Rodabough RJ, *et al.* Effect of estrogen therapy on gallbladder disease. *JAMA* 2005;293:330–9

Hulley S, Grady D, Bush T, *et al.* Randomized trial of estrogen plus progestin for secondary prevention of coronary heart disease in postmenopausal women. Heart and Estrogen/progestin Replacement Study (HERS) Research Group. *JAMA* 1998;**280**:605–13.

Cardiovascular disease (coronary heart disease (CHD) and stroke)

Alexander KP, Newby LK, Hellkamp AS, *et al.* Initiation of hormone replacement therapy after acute myocardial infarction is associated with more cardiac events during follow-up. *J Am Coll Cardiol* 2001;**38**:1–7.

Angerer P, Stork S, Kothny W, *et al.* Effect of oral postmenopausal hormone replacement on progression of atherosclerosis: a randomized, controlled trial. *Arterioscler Thromb Vasc Biol* 2001;**21**:262–8.

Cherry N, Gilmour K, Hannaford P, *et al.* Oestrogen therapy for prevention of reinfarction in postmenopausal women: a randomised placebo controlled trial. *Lancet* 2002;**360**:2001–8.

Clarke SC, Kelleher J, Lloyd-Jones H, *et al.* A study of hormone replacement therapy in postmenopausal women with ischaemic heart disease: the Papworth HRT atherosclerosis study. *Br J Obstet Gynaecol* 2002;**109**:1056–62.

Clarkson TB, Appt SE. Controversies about HRT – lessons from monkey models. *Maturitas* 2005;**51**:64–74.

Gabriel SR, Carmona L, Roque M, *et al.* Hormone replacement therapy for preventing cardiovascular disease in post-menopausal women. *Cochrane Database Syst Rev* 2005;(2):CD002229.

Grodstein F, Manson JE, Colditz GA, *et al.* A prospective, observational study of postmenopausal hormone therapy and primary prevention of cardiovascular disease. *Ann Intern Med* 2000;**133**:933–41.

Grodstein F, Manson JE, Stampfer MJ. Postmenopausal hormone use and secondary prevention of coronary events in the Nurses' Health Study. A prospective, observational study. *Ann Intern Med* 2001;**135**:1–8.

Grodstein F, Stampfer MJ, Colditz GA, *et al.* Postmenopausal hormone therapy and mortality. *N Engl J Med* 1997;**336**:1769–75.

Herrington DM, Reboussin DM, Brosnihan KB, *et al.* Effects of estrogen replacement on the progression of coronary-artery atherosclerosis. *N Engl J Med* 2000; **343**:522–9.

Hulley S, Grady D, Bush T, *et al.* Randomized trial of estrogen plus progestin for secondary prevention of coronary heart disease in postmenopausal women. Heart and Estrogen/progestin Replacement Study (HERS) Research Group. *JAMA* 1998;**280**:605–13.

Manson JE, Hsia J, Johnson KC, *et al.*, Women's Health Initiative Investigators. Estrogen plus progestin and the risk of coronary heart disease. *N Engl J Med* 2003; **349**:523–34.

Newton KM, LaCroix AZ, McKnight B, *et al.* Estrogen replacement therapy and prognosis after first myocardial infarction. *Am J Epidemiol* 1997;**145**:269–77.

Petitti DB, Sidney S, Quesenberry CP Jr, Bernstein A. Ischemic stroke and use of estrogen and estrogen/progestogen as hormone replacement therapy. *Stroke* 1998;**29**:23–8.

Psaty BM, Heckbert SR, Atkins D, *et al.* The risk of myocardial infarction associated with the combined use of estrogens and progestins in postmenopausal women. *Arch Intern Med* 1994;**154**:1333–9.

Shlipak MG, Angeja BG, Go AS, *et al.* Hormone therapy and in-hospital survival after myocardial infarction in postmenopausal women. *Circulation* 2001;**104**:2300–4.

Shlipak MG, Simon JA, Vittinghoff E, *et al.* Estrogen and progestin, lipoprotein(a), and the risk of recurrent coronary heart disease events after menopause. *JAMA* 2000;**283**:1845–52.

Simon JA, Hsia J, Cauley JA, *et al.* Postmenopausal hormone therapy and risk of stroke: The Heart and Estrogen-progestin Replacement Study (HERS). *Circulation* 2001;**103**:638–42.

The Women's Health Initiative Steering Committee. Effects of conjugated equine estrogen in postmenopausal women with hysterectomy: the Women's Health Initiative randomized controlled trial. *JAMA* 2004;**291**:1701–12.

van Baal WM, Emeis JJ, van der Mooren MJ, *et al.* Impaired procoagulant-anticoagulant balance during hormone replacement therapy? A randomised, placebo-controlled 12-week study. *Thromb Haemost* 2000;**83**:29–34.

Viscoli CM, Brass LM, Kernan WN, *et al.* A clinical trial of estrogen-replacement therapy after ischemic stroke. *N Engl J Med* 2001;**345**:1243–9.

Wassertheil-Smoller S, Hendrix SL, Limacher M, *et al.* Effect of estrogen plus progestin on stroke in postmenopausal women: the Women's Health Initiative: a randomized trial. *JAMA* 2003;**289**:2673–84.

Dementia and cognition

Baldereschi M, Di Carlo A, Lepore V, *et al.* Estrogen-replacement therapy and Alzheimer's disease in the Italian Longitudinal Study on Aging. *Neurology* 1998;**50**:996–1002.

Espeland MA, Rapp SR, Shumaker SA, *et al.* Conjugated equine estrogens and global cognitive function in postmenopausal women: Women's Health Initiative Memory Study. *JAMA* 2004;**291**:2959–68.

Henderson VW, Paganini-Hill A, Miller BL, *et al.* Estrogen for Alzheimer's disease in women: randomized, double-blind, placebo-controlled trial. *Neurology* 2000; **54**:295–301.

Kesslak JP. Can estrogen play a significant role in the prevention of Alzheimer's disease? *J Neural Transm Suppl* 2002;**62**:227–39.

de Moraes SA, Szklo M, Knopman D, Park E. Prospective assessment of estrogen replacement therapy and cognitive functioning: atherosclerosis risk in communities study. *Am J Epidemiol* 2001;**154**:733–9.

Mulnard RA, Cotman CW, Kawas C, *et al.* Estrogen replacement therapy for treatment of mild to moderate Alzheimer disease: a randomized controlled trial. Alzheimer's Disease Cooperative Study. *JAMA* 2000;**283**:1007–15.

Paganini-Hill A, Henderson VW. Estrogen replacement therapy and risk of Alzheimer's disease. *Arch Intern Med* 1996;**156**:2213–17.

Rapp SR, Espeland MA, Shumaker SA, *et al.* Effect of estrogen plus progestin on global cognitive function in postmenopausal women: The Women's Health Initiative Memory Study: a randomized controlled trial. *JAMA* 2003;**289**:2663–72.

Shaywitz SE, Shaywitz BA, Pugh KR, *et al.* Effect of estrogen on brain activation patterns in postmenopausal women during working memory tasks. *JAMA* 1999;**281**:1197–202.

Shumaker SA, Legault C, Kuller L, *et al.*; Women's Health Initiative Memory Study. Conjugated equine estrogens and incidence of probable dementia and mild cognitive impairment in postmenopausal women: Women's Health Initiative Memory Study. *JAMA* 2004;**291**:2947–58.

Shumaker SA, Legault C, Rapp SR, *et al.* Estrogen plus progestin and the incidence of dementia and mild cognitive impairment in postmenopausal women: the Women's Health Initiative Memory Study: a randomized controlled trial. *JAMA* 2003; **289**:2651–62.

Viscoli CM, Brass LM, Kernan WN, *et al.* Estrogen therapy and risk of cognitive decline: results from the Women's Estrogen for Stroke Trial (WEST). *Am J Obstet Gynecol* 2005;**192**:387–93.

Wang PN, Liao SQ, Liu RS, *et al.* Effects of estrogen on cognition, mood, and cerebral blood flow in AD: a controlled study. *Neurology* 2000;**54**:2061–6.

Zandi PP, Carlson MC, Plassman BL, *et al.* Hormone replacement therapy and incidence of Alzheimer disease in older women: the Cache County Study. *JAMA* 2002;**288**:2123–9.

Ovarian cancer

Anderson GL, Judd HL, Kaunitz AM, *et al.*; Women's Health Initiative Investigators. Effects of estrogen plus progestin on gynecologic cancers and associated diagnostic procedures: the Women's Health Initiative randomized trial. *JAMA* 2003; **290**:1739–48.

Garg PP, Kerlikowske K, Subak L, Grady D. Hormone replacement therapy and the risk of epithelial ovarian carcinoma: a meta-analysis. *Obstet Gynecol* 1998;**92**:472–9.

Negri E, Tzonou A, Beral V, *et al.* Hormonal therapy for menopause and ovarian cancer in a collaborative re-analysis of European studies. *Int J Cancer* 1999; **80**:848–51.

Persson I, Yuen J, Bergkvist L, Schairer C. Cancer incidence and mortality in women receiving estrogen and estrogen-progestin replacement therapy – long-term follow-up of a Swedish cohort. *Int J Cancer* 1996;**67**:327–32.

Riman T. Hormone replacement therapy and epithelial ovarian cancer: is there an association? *J Br Menopause Soc* 2003;**9**:61–8.

Rodriguez C, Patel AV, Calle EE, *et al.* Estrogen replacement therapy and ovarian cancer mortality in a large prospective study of US women. *JAMA* 2001;**285**:1460–5.

Quality of life

Brunner RL, Gass M, Aragaki A, *et al.*; Women's Health Initiative Investigators. Effects of conjugated equine estrogen on health-related quality of life in postmenopausal women with hysterectomy: results from the Women's Health Initiative Randomized Clinical Trial. *Arch Intern Med* 2005;**165**:1976–86.

Hays J, Ockene JK, Brunner RL, *et al.* Effects of estrogen plus progestin on health-related quality of life. *N Engl J Med* 2003;**348**:1839–54.

Zethraeus N, Johannesson M, Henriksson P, Strand RT. The impact of hormone replacement therapy on quality of life and willingness to pay. *Br J Obstet Gynaecol* 1997;**104**:1191–5.

8 Non-oestrogen-based treatments for menopausal symptoms and osteoporosis

Menopausal symptoms
Prevention and treatment of osteoporosis
Further reading

Menopausal symptoms

Hot flushes

Progestogens

Progestogens such as 5 mg/day norethisterone or 40 mg/day megestrol acetate can be effective in controlling hot flushes and night sweats. At such doses, norethisterone affords some limited protection of the skeleton, but, at present, no data exist about megestrol acetate. Furthermore, at doses that achieve control of vasomotor symptoms, the risk of venous thromboembolism is increased.

Clonidine

Clonidine is a centrally acting α-adrenoceptor agonist that was developed originally for the treatment of hypertension. A dose of 50–75 mg twice daily has limited value and effectiveness.

Selective serotonin reuptake inhibitors and serotonin and noradrenaline reuptake inhibitors

Short-term studies show that paroxetine, fluoxetine, citalopram and venlafaxine are effective in treating hot flushes and increase the range of options when oestrogen is contraindicated. Their efficacy has been questioned in longer studies, however, and there are concerns about safety and addiction.

Gabapentin

Gabapentin is a gamma-aminobutyric acid analogue used to treat epilepsy, neurogenic pain and migraine. Limited evidence shows that it may be effective.

Propranolol
Propranolol should not be used now, because studies of its effects have produced conflicting results.

Vaginal atrophy

Traditional lubricants and newer vaginal moisturizers are available without prescription. Published data about scientific trials are limited.

Lubricants
Lubricants generally are considered to be temporary measures to relieve vaginal dryness during intercourse. Their formulations are a combination of protectants and thickening agents in a water-soluble base. Short durations of action limit their usefulness as a long-term solution. Lubricants must be applied frequently for more continuous relief and require reapplication before sexual activity.

The integrity and efficacy of condoms may be compromised by lubricants such as petroleum-based products and baby oil. This is important when condoms are used to prevent sexually transmitted infections (see Chapter 4).

Moisturizers
Moisturizers claim to provide more than transient lubrication. Formulations may include a bioadhesive polycarbophil-based polymer, which attaches to mucin and epithelial cells on the vaginal wall and retains water. Moisturizers are promoted as providing long-term relief of vaginal dryness (rather than being just sexual aids) and need to be applied less frequently. Currently, one moisturizer in the UK is available on prescription.

Prevention and treatment of osteoporosis

Pharmacological interventions

All pharmacological interventions except for parathyroid hormone and strontium ranelate act mainly by inhibiting bone resorption (Table 8.1). Most of the studies have been undertaken in postmenopausal women with osteoporosis or at increased risk of the disease, and information in perimenopausal women or those with premature ovarian failure are scant. Very few data exist about long-term efficacy for reducing fractures (that is, more than 10 years of treatment) and safety of combinations of therapy. In many of the studies, the placebo group received calcium and vitamin D supplements.

Table 8.1

Interventions for the prevention and treatment of osteoporosis

	Spine	Hip
Bisphosphonates		
Etidronate	A	B
Alendronate	A	A
Risedronate	A	A
Ibandronate	A	ND
Calcitrol	A	ND
Calcitonin	A	B
Selective oestrogen receptor modulators (SERMs)	A	ND
Strontium ranelate	A	A
Teriparatide (parathyroid hormone)	A	ND

ND = not demonstrated

The levels of evidence for the various agents detailed are:

A = Meta-analysis of randomized controlled trials (RCTs) or from at least one RCT or from at least one well-designed controlled study without randomization

B = From at least one other type of well-designed quasi-experimental study or from well-designed non-experimental descriptive studies, eg comparative studies, correlation studies and case–control studies

Bisphosphonates

Alendronate, risedronate, etidronate and ibandronate are used in the prevention and treatment of osteoporosis. The first three are also used in corticosteroid-induced osteoporosis, and limited data suggest that they seem to have a synergistic effect on bone density in combination with oestrogen, and gain in bone mineral density (BMD) is greater than that achieved by either agent alone.

Bisphosphonates are chemical analogues of pyrophosphate that began life as agents to remove calcium deposits in pipes and washing machines. The replacement of a P–O–P bond with a P–C–P bond results in a stable compound resistant to degradation by pyrophosphatases that occur naturally in the body.

Bisphosphonates can be classified into two groups:

- non-nitrogen containing bisphosphonates, such as etidronate
- nitrogen-containing bisphosphonates, such as alendronate, risedronate and ibandronate.

All bisphosphonates are absorbed poorly from the gastrointestinal tract and must be given on an empty stomach. Food or calcium-containing drinks (except water) inhibit the absorption, which at best is only 5–10% of the administered dose. The principal side-effect of all bisphosphonates is irritation of the upper gastrointestinal tract. Symptoms resolve quickly after drug withdrawal and these adverse effects are much reduced by using weekly or monthly rather than daily regimens.

Alendronate

Alendronate is an aminobisphosphonate that reduces vertebral and non-vertebral fractures by 50% in randomized controlled trials. Multiple long-term studies have shown that it maintains and increases BMD of the hip and spine in postmenopausal women. Changes are most marked in the first year, but BMD continues to increase up to at least 10 years of treatment and seems to be maintained for at least two years after the drug is stopped. The dose for prevention of osteoporosis is 5 mg/day or 35 mg once weekly and for the treatment of established disease is 10 mg/day or 70 mg once weekly.

Risedronate

Risedronate is a pyridinyl bisphosphonate that also reduces vertebral and non-vertebral fractures in randomized controlled trials. The antifracture effect of risedronate continues after at least seven years of treatment. The dose for treatment of established disease is 5 mg/day or 35 mg once weekly.

Ibandronate

Ibandronate is an aminobisphosphonate that reduces vertebral but not non-vertebral fractures by 50% in randomized controlled trials undertaken in postmenopausal women. It was licensed in 2005 for the prevention and treatment of osteoporosis, and the dose is 2.5 mg/day or 150 mg once monthly.

Etidronate

Etidronate was the first bisphosphonate to be developed. It is given intermittently (400 mg on 14 of every 90 days), and 1250 mg of calcium salts are given during the remaining 76 days. Although data from randomized controlled trials are available for vertebral fracture, none are available for non-vertebral fracture.

The question of how long to prescribe a bisphosphonate has not been fully clarified yet, because of concerns about 'frozen bone', with complete turning off of bone remodelling with long-term use and also development of osteonecrosis in the jaw. The biological model of frozen bone is osteopetrosis: a heterogeneous group of heritable conditions in which a defect in bone resorption by osteoclasts exists, BMD is high and bone is brittle. Delayed and absent healing of spontaneous non-spinal fractures has been reported in patients treated with alendronate, with biopsies showing suppression of the formation of new bone. Five years of treatment with a two-year 'holiday' have been proposed for alendronate, but differences may exist with individual bisphosphonates. This may not be applicable to glucocorticoid-induced osteoporosis. Concerns also exist about the use of bisphosphonates in perimenopausal women, as most data will have been obtained in older women with osteoporosis or at risk of the disease. Limited data have shown stabilization of bone density with alendronate but no difference in the rate of fractures compared with placebo.

Comparisons have been made between alendronate and risedronate and between alendronate and raloxifene, but so far they have been limited to their effects on BMD rather than the risk of fracture.

Selective oestrogen receptor modulators

Compounds that possess oestrogenic actions in certain tissues and anti-oestrogenic actions in others are described as selective (o)estrogen receptor modulators (SERMs). By offering the opportunity to target antagonist or agonist activity on specific tissues, SERMs may have significant potential for the treatment and prevention of important diseases, including breast cancer, osteoporosis and cardiovascular disease.

The non-steroidal anti-oestrogen tamoxifen was one of the first SERMs. As it behaves as an oestrogen antagonist in the breast, it is used as an adjuvant treatment for breast cancer; however, it was also found to display beneficial oestrogen agonist-like effects on bone and lipids, but it has no licence for use in osteoporosis. Concerns also exist about the adverse effects of tamoxifen on the endometrium, where it acts as an oestrogen and increases the risk of endometrial hyperplasia and cancer.

Raloxifene is licensed for the prevention of osteoporosis-related vertebral fracture. It reduces vertebral fracture by 30–50%, depending on the dose, in women with established osteoporosis; however, there is as yet no evidence of efficacy in non-vertebral fracture, such as fracture of the hip. Raloxifene taken in a dose of 60 mg/day is associated with some transient side-effects, such as vasomotor flushes and calf cramps. Raloxifene does not treat the symptoms of the menopause and is therefore not suitable for women with hot flushes. It does, however, share with conventional hormone replacement therapy (HRT) an equal propensity to cause venous thromboembolism.

The clinical advantage of raloxifene is that it achieves bone protection without stimulating the endometrium or the breast. Thus patients are amenorrhoeic and do not complain of breast tenderness. Indeed, raloxifene reduces the risk of breast cancer in women with osteoporosis. It also reduces levels of total cholesterol and LDL-C and thus may be cardioprotective. The Raloxifene Use for the Heart (RUTH) Study, and the Study of Tamoxifen and

Raloxifene are examining the role of raloxifene in coronary heart disease and in the prevention of breast cancer.

At a dose of 120 mg/day, but not 60 mg/day, raloxifene reduces the risk of cognitive impairment in postmenopausal women with osteoporosis. With regard to the lower genital tract, it does not seem to have any oestrogenic effects, does not increase the incidence of urinary incontinence compared with placebo and may worsen prolapse.

In asymptomatic postmenopausal women with significant risk of vertebral fracture, raloxifene, therefore, is likely to play a major role in women who cannot or will not take HRT and who are generally aged 60–75 years.

Parathyroid hormone

Although hyperparathyroidism is associated with bone loss, the interaction between the peptide parathyroid hormone (PTH), which contains 84 amino acids, and the skeleton is more complex than was initially thought. Although continuous or tonic production of PTH does promote osteoclastic bone resorption, pulsed or clonic release of hormone seems to have precisely the opposite effect. Teriparatide (human PTH(1–34) recombinant origin) is identical in its sequence of amino acids to the biologically active portion of the native hormone(1–34). In a pivotal study undertaken in 1637 postmenopausal women with previous vertebral fractures, teriparatide significantly decreased the risk of vertebral but not hip fractures. The dose of 40 µg increased BMD more than the dose of 20 µg but had similar effects on the risk of fracture and was more likely to have side-effects. It is used in cases of severe osteoporosis, with 20 µg administered daily by subcutaneous injection for 18 months. No synergy between PTH and alendronate has been found. Indeed, results suggest that the concurrent use of alendronate may reduce the anabolic effects of PTH. Conversely, synergy has been found with oestrogen.

Strontium ranelate

Strontium was originally detected in lead mines near Strontian, Scotland, in the late 1700s. Like calcium, it is an alkaline earth element (from Group II in the periodic table as are magnesium, barium and radium). It is present in water and food and in trace amounts throughout the skeleton. Although absorption is poor when strontium is consumed orally, calcified tissues and areas of active osteogenesis take up 50–80% of the absorbed dose. Because of its bone-seeking properties, strontium was used widely in the 1950s for the management of osteoporosis, but it fell out of favour because mineralization defects were observed and the synthesis of calcitriol was inhibited. These adverse effects were thought possibly to have been due to calcium-deficient diets and the doses used, and interest in developing this old element as a new compound, strontium ranelate, has been renewed. Randomized controlled trials have shown a decreased risk of vertebral and hip fractures with strontium ranelate. A 2 g sachet is administered daily, with the sachet's contents dissolved in water; it should be taken at least two hours after food. The most common side-effects are mild and transient nausea and diarrhoea but are rare in absolute terms.

Calcitriol
This is the active metabolite of vitamin D and facilitates the intestinal absorption of calcium. It also has direct effects on bone cells. Studies of the effects of calcitriol on bone loss and fractures have produced conflicting results, mainly because of small sample sizes. The largest study had a single-blind design and involved 622 postmenopausal women. The placebo group of women, who received calcium alone, showed an increasing rate of new vertebral fractures, whereas the calcitriol group showed no change in the rate of vertebral fractures. Bone mineral density was not measured. A decrease was also seen in the rate of non-vertebral fractures. That the rate of fracture in women who took calcium should have increased is bizarre. The potential dangers of hypercalcaemia and hypercalciuria mean that levels of calcium in serum and urine should be monitored closely, so its use is limited.

Calcitonin
Calcitonin can be given by subcutaneous or intramuscular injection or by nasal spray. Parenteral calcitonin is expensive, produces side-effects such as nausea, diarrhoea and flushing and results in the production of neutralizing antibodies in some patients. Nasal calcitonin has also been shown to reduce new vertebral fractures in women with established osteoporosis. Evidence exists for its efficacy as an analgesic in acute vertebral fracture. It may also be helpful as an adjunctive treatment after surgery for hip fracture. An oral preparation is being developed.

Future developments
The suggestion that statins may reduce the risk of osteoporotic fracture has not been supported so far in randomized controlled trials. The efficacy of fluoride regimens is unproved, and their use for the treatment of osteoporosis is currently not recommended. Bisphosphonates with a yearly dose schedule, new SERMs and drugs such as denosumab (AMG 162) which target osteoprotegerin and RANKL involved in bone remodelling are likely to appear.

Non-pharmacological interventions: calcium and vitamin D

Supplementation with calcium and vitamin D particularly may be relevant when much evidence of insufficiency exists, especially in elderly people.

Table 8.2

Calcium content of some foods

Food	Calcium content (mg)
Full-fat milk (250 ml)	295
Semi-skimmed milk (250 ml)	300
Skimmed milk (250 ml)	305
Low-fat yogurt (100 g)	150
Cheddar cheese (50 g)	360
Boiled spinach (100 g)	159
Brazil nuts (100 g)	170
Tinned salmon (100 g)	93
Tofu (100 g)	480

Whatever treatment is used to prevent or treat osteoporosis, an essential part of the management is the provision of adequate dietary or supplemental calcium and vitamin D. In northern latitudes, the cutaneous synthesis of vitamin D occurs only in the summer months, and the national diet in the UK lacks sufficient amounts of this vitamin for adequate intake in the absence of solar exposure (Table 8.2). Other countries, such as the US, fortify foods by adding vitamin D to dairy products.

Most studies show that about 1.5 g of elemental calcium is necessary to preserve bone health in postmenopausal women and elderly women who are not taking HRT. This figure has been reinforced recently, although current recommendations in the UK of 700 mg/day are unlikely to change. In women who use HRT, 1 g/day is sufficient to maintain calcium balance.

The effects of calcium and vitamin D supplements alone or in combination on fracture, however, are contradictory. This may depend on the study population. People in sheltered accommodation or residential care may be more frail, have lower dietary intakes of calcium and vitamin D and are at higher risk of fracture than those living in the community. There are concerns about vitamin D status on bone gain in adolescence: pubertal girls with hypovitaminosis D seem to be at risk of not reaching maximum peak bone mass, particularly at the lumbar spine.

Calcium

A meta-analysis of 15 trials representing 1806 participants showed that calcium was more effective than placebo in reducing rates of bone loss after two or more years of treatment. The pooled difference in percentage change from baseline was 2.05% (0.24% to 3.86%) for total body bone density, 1.66% (0.92% to 2.39%) for the lumbar spine at two years, 1.60% (0.78% to 2.41%) for the hip and 1.91% (0.33% to 3.50%) for the distal radius. The relative risk of fractures of the vertebrae was 0.79% (0.54% to 1.09%) and of non-vertebral fractures was 0.86% (0.43% to 1.72%). Thus calcium supplementation alone has a small positive effect on bone density. The data show a trend towards a reduction in vertebral fractures, but whether calcium reduces the incidence of non-vertebral fractures is unclear. Furthermore, no evidence shows that calcium supplements can reverse bone loss in the perimenopause.

Vitamin D
Vitamin D exposure has been reported to reduce the risk of fracture and falls, but, again, the evidence is conflicting. A meta-analysis of 12 randomized controlled trials involving 19,314 participants found that a dose of vitamin D of 700–800 IU/day reduced the relative risk (RR) of hip fracture by 26% (RR 0.74 (0.61 to 0.88)) and any non-vertebral fracture by 23% (RR 0.77 (0.68 to 0.87)) versus calcium or placebo. No significant benefit was observed for RCTs that used 400 IU/day vitamin D (RR for hip fracture 1.15 (0.88 to 1.50); RR for any non-vertebral fracture 1.03 (0.86 to 1.24)). The authors thus concluded that oral supplementation of vitamin D at a dose of 700–800 IU/day seems to reduce the risk of hip and any non-vertebral fractures in ambulatory or institutionalized elderly people. An oral dose of vitamin D of 400 IU/day is not sufficient for fracture prevention.

Calcium and vitamin D
Calcium and vitamin D exposure has also been reported to reduce the risk of fracture, but, again, the evidence is conflicting. An early French study had shown a 30% lower risk of hip fracture in elderly women given 1.2 g of elemental calcium and 800 IU of vitamin D. Bone mineral density at the hip increased, and secondary hyperparathyroidism present in many women at the outset was reversed in the active treatment group but continued in the placebo group. A significant reduction was also seen in all long bone fractures in women treated for 18 months. More recent studies in community dwelling women or as a secondary prevention, however, show no benefit.

Further reading
Menopausal symptoms

Barton DL, Loprinzi CL, Novotny P, *et al.* Pilot evaluation of citalopram for the relief of hot flashes. *J Support Oncol* 2003;1:47–51.

Bygdeman M, Swahn ML. Replens versus dienoestrol cream in the symptomatic treatment of vaginal atrophy in postmenopausal women. *Maturitas* 1996;23:259–63.

Committee on Safety of Medicines. *Selective Serotonin Reuptake Inhibitor (SSRI) Antidepressants – Findings of the Committee on Safety of Medicines (CSM).* London: Committee on Safety of Medicines, 2004.

David A, Don R, Tajchner G, Weissglas L. Veralipride: alternative antidopaminergic treatment for menopausal symptoms. *Am J Obstet Gynecol* 1988;**158**:1107–111.

Guttuso T Jr, Kurlan R, McDermott MP, Kieburtz K. Gabapentin's effects on hot flashes in postmenopausal women: a randomized controlled trial. *Obstet Gynecol* 2003;**101**:337–45.

Loprinzi CL, Kugler JW, Sloan JA, *et al.* Venlafaxine in management of hot flashes in survivors of breast cancer: a randomised controlled trial. *Lancet* 2000;**356**:2059–63.

Pandya KJ, Morrow GR, Roscoe JA, *et al.* Gabapentin for hot flashes in 420 women with breast cancer: a randomised double-blind placebo-controlled trial. *Lancet* 2005;**366**:818–24.

Pandya KJ, Raubertas RF, Flynn PJ, *et al.* Oral clonidine in postmenopausal patients with breast cancer experiencing tamoxifen-induced hot flashes: a University of Rochester Cancer Center Community Clinical Oncology Program study. *Ann Intern Med* 2000;**132**:788–93.

Rees M, Mander T. *Managing the Menopause without Oestrogen.* London: RSM Press, 2004.

Rosen AD, Rosen T. Study of condom integrity after brief exposure to over-the-counter vaginal preparations. *South Med J* 1999;**92**:305–7.

Stearns V, Isaacs C, Rowland J, *et al.* A pilot trial assessing the efficacy of paroxetine hydrochloride (Paxil) in controlling hot flashes in breast cancer survivors. *Ann Oncol* 2000;**11**:17–22.

Suvanto-Luukkonen E, Koivunen R, Sundstrom H, *et al.* Citalopram and fluoxetine in the treatment of postmenopausal symptoms: a prospective, randomized, 9-month, placebo-controlled, double-blind study. *Menopause* 2005;**12**:18–26.

Vasilakis C, Jick H, del Mar Melero-Montes M. Risk of idiopathic venous thromboembolism in users of progestogens alone. *Lancet* 1999;**354**:1610–11.

Willhite LA, O'Connell MB. Urogenital atrophy: prevention and treatment. *Pharmacotherapy* 2001;**21**:464–80.

Osteoporosis general references

Royal College of Physicians. *Osteoporosis: Clinical Guidelines for Prevention and Treatment.* London: Royal College of Physicians, 1999. http://www.rcplondon.ac.uk/ (last accessed 29 September 2005).

Royal College of Physicians. *Osteoporosis: Clinical Guidelines for Prevention and Treatment. Update on Pharmacological Interventions and an Algorithm for Management.* London: Royal College of Physicians, 2000. http://www.rcplondon.ac.uk/ (last accessed 29 September 2005).

Bisphosphonates

Bone HG, Greenspan SL, McKeever C, *et al.* Alendronate and estrogen effects in postmenopausal women with low bone mineral density. Alendronate/Estrogen Study Group. *J Clin Endocrinol Metab* 2000;**85**:720–6.

Chesnut CH III, Skag A, Christiansen C, *et al.* Effects of oral ibandronate administered daily or intermittently on fracture risk in postmenopausal osteoporosis. *J Bone Miner Res* 2004;**19**:1241–9.

Cranney A, Guyatt G, Krolicki B, *et al.* A meta-analysis of etidronate for the treatment of postmenopausal osteoporosis. *Osteoporos Int* 2001;**12**:140–51.

Delmas PD, Recker RR, Chesnut CH 3rd, *et al.* Daily and intermittent oral ibandronate normalize bone turnover and provide significant reduction in vertebral fracture risk: results from the BONE study. *Osteoporos Int* 2004;**15**:792–8.

Emkey R, Reid I, Mulloy A, *et al.* Ten-year efficacy and safety of alendronate in the treatment of osteoporosis in postmenopausal women. *J Bone Miner Res* 2002; **17**:S319.

Harris ST, Eriksen EF, Davidson M, *et al.* Effect of combined risedronate and hormone replacement therapies on bone mineral density in postmenopausal women. *J Clin Endocrinol Metab* 2001;**86**:1890–7.

Harris ST, Watts NB, Genant HK, *et al.* Effects of risedronate treatment on vertebral and nonvertebral fractures in women with postmenopausal osteoporosis. *JAMA* 1999;**282**:1344–52.

Hosking D, Adami S, Felsenberg D, *et al.* Comparison of change in bone resorption and bone mineral density with once-weekly alendronate and daily risedronate: a randomised, placebo-controlled study. *Curr Med Res Opin* 2003;**19**:383–94.

Luckey M, Kagan R, Greenspan S, *et al.* Once-weekly alendronate 70 mg and raloxifene 60 mg daily in the treatment of postmenopausal osteoporosis. *Menopause* 2004;**11**:405–15.

McClung MR, Geusens P, Miller MD, *et al.* Effect of risedronate on the risk of hip fracture in elderly women. *N Engl J Med* 2001;**344**:333–40.

Miller PD, McClung MR, Macovei L, *et al.* Monthly oral ibandronate therapy in postmenopausal osteoporosis: 1-year results from the MOBILE study. *J Bone Miner Res* 2005;**20**:1315–22.

Odvina CV, Zerwekh JE, Rao DS, *et al.* Severely suppressed bone turnover: a potential complication of alendronate therapy. *J Clin Endocrinol Metab* 2005;**90**:1294–301.

Ravn P, Bidstrup M, Wasnich RD, *et al.* Alendronate and estrogen-progestin in the long-term prevention of bone loss: four-year results from the early postmenopausal intervention cohort study. A randomized, controlled trial. *Ann Intern Med* 1999;**131**:935–42.

Reginster JY, Wilson KM, Dumont E, *et al.* Monthly oral ibandronate is well tolerated and efficacious in postmenopausal women: results from the monthly oral pilot study. *J Clin Endocrinol Metab* 2005;**90**:5018–24.

Reid DM, Hughes RA, Laan RF, *et al.* Efficacy and safety of daily risedronate in the treatment of corticosteroid-induced osteoporosis in men and women: a randomized trial. European Corticosteroid-Induced Osteoporosis Treatment Study. *J Bone Miner Res* 2000;**15**:1006–13

Rosen CJ, Hochberg MC, Bonnick SL, *et al.* Treatment with once-weekly alendronate 70 mg compared with once-weekly risedronate 35 mg in women with postmenopausal osteoporosis: a randomized double-blind study. *J Bone Miner Res* 2005;**20**:141–51

Ruggiero SL, Mehrotra B, Rosenberg TJ, Engroff SL. Osteonecrosis of the jaws associated with the use of bisphosphonates: a review of 63 cases. *J Oral Maxillofac Surg* 2004;**62**:527–34.

Schnitzer T, Bone HG, Crepaldi G, *et al.* Alendronate 70 mg once weekly is therapeutically equivalent to alendronate 10 mg daily for the treatment of postmenopausal osteoporosis. *Aging Clin Exp Res* 2000;**12**:1–12.

Sebba AI, Bonnick SL, Kagan R, *et al.* Response to therapy with once-weekly alendronate 70 mg compared to once-weekly risedronate 35 mg in the treatment of postmenopausal osteoporosis. *Curr Med Res Opin* 2004;**20**:2031–41.

Sorensen OH, Crawford GM, Mulder H, *et al.* Long-term efficacy of risedronate: a 5-year placebo-controlled clinical experience. *Bone* 2003;**32**:120–6.

Tolar J, Teitelbaum SL, Orchard PJ. Osteopetrosis. *N Engl J Med* 2004;**351**:2839–49.

Selective oestrogen receptor modulators

Cauley JA, Norton L, Lippman ME, *et al.* Continued breast cancer risk reduction in postmenopausal women treated with raloxifene: 4-year results from the MORE trial. *Breast Cancer Res Treat* 2001;**65**:125–32.

Cosman F, Baz-Hecht M, Cushman M, *et al.* Short-term effects of estrogen, tamoxifen and raloxifene on hemostasis: a randomized-controlled study and review of the literature. *Thromb Res* 2005;**116**:1–13.

Delmas PD, Genant HK, Crans GG, *et al.* Severity of prevalent vertebral fractures and the risk of subsequent vertebral and nonverterbral fractures: results from the MORE trial. *Bone* 2003;**33**:522–32.

Ettinger B, Black DM, Mitlak BH, *et al.* Reduction of vertebral fracture risk in postmenopausal women with osteoporosis treated with raloxifene. *JAMA* 1999;**282**:637–45.

Goldstein SR, Neven P, Zhou L, *et al.* Raloxifene effect on frequency of surgery for pelvic floor relaxation. *Obstet Gynecol* 2001;**98**:91–6.

Goldstein SR, Johnson S, Watts NB, *et al.* Incidence of urinary incontinence in postmenopausal women treated with raloxifene or estrogen. *Menopause* 2005;**12**:160–4.

Jolly E, Bjarnason NH, Neven P, *et al.* Prevention of osteoporosis and uterine effects in postmenopausal women taking raloxifene for 5 years. *Menopause* 2003;**10**:337–44.

Keech CA, Sashegyi A, Barrett-Connor E. Year-by-year analysis of cardiovascular events in the Multiple Outcomes of Raloxifene Evaluation (MORE) trial. *Curr Med Res Opin* 2005;**21**:135–40.

Riggs BL, Melton LJ. Bone turnover matters: the raloxifene treatment paradox of dramatic decreases in vertebral fractures without commensurate increases in bone density. *J Bone Miner Res* 2002;**17**:11–14.

Siris ES, Harris ST, Eastell R, *et al.* Skeletal effects of raloxifene after 8 years: results from the Continuing Outcomes Relevant to Evista (CORE) Study. *J Bone Miner Res* 2005;**20**:1514–24.

Vardy MB, Lindsay R, Scotti RJ, *et al.* Short-term urogenital effects of raloxifene, tamoxifen, and estrogen. *Am J Obstet Gynecol* 2003;**189**:81–8.

Yaffe K, Krueger K, Cummings SR, *et al.* Effect of raloxifene on prevention of dementia and cognitive impairment in older women: the Multiple Outcomes of Raloxifene Evaluation (MORE) randomized trial. *Am J Psychiatry* 2005;**162**:683–90.

Parathyroid hormone and strontium ranelate

Black DM, Greenspan SL, Ensrud KE, *et al.* The effects of parathyroid hormone and alendronate alone or in combination in postmenopausal osteoporosis. *N Engl J Med* 2003;**349**:1207–15.

Cosman F, Nieves J, Woelfert L, *et al.* Parathyroid hormone added to established hormone therapy: effects on vertebral fracture and maintenance of bone mass after parathyroid hormone withdrawal. *J Bone Miner Res* 2001;**16**:925–31.

El-Hajj Fuleihan G. Strontium ranelate – a novel therapy for osteoporosis or a permutation of the same? *N Engl J Med* 2004;**350**:504–6.

Meunier PJ, Roux C, Seeman E, *et al.* The effects of strontium ranelate on the risk of vertebral fracture in women with postmenopausal osteoporosis. *N Engl J Med* 2004;**350**:459–68.

Neer RM, Arnaud CD, Zanchetta JR, *et al.* Effect of parathyroid hormone (1-34) on fractures and bone mineral density in postmenopausal women with osteoporosis. *N Engl J Med* 2001;**344**:1434–41.

Reginster JY, Seeman E, De Vernejoul MC, *et al.* Strontium ranelate reduces the risk of nonvertebral fractures in postmenopausal women with osteoporosis: Treatment of Peripheral Osteoporosis (TROPOS) Study. *J Clin Endocrinol Metab* 2005;**90**:2816–22.

Calcitriol and calcitonin

Chapuy MC, Arlot ME, Duboeuf F, *et al.* Vitamin D3 and calcium to prevent hip fractures in elderly women. *N Engl J Med* 1992;**327**:1637–42.

Chesnut CH 3rd, Silverman S, Andriano K, *et al.* A randomized trial of nasal spray salmon calcitonin in postmenopausal women with established osteoporosis: the prevent recurrence of osteoporotic fractures study. PROOF Study Group. *Am J Med* 2000;**109**:267–76.

Huusko TM, Karppi P, Kautiainen H, *et al.* Randomized, double-blind, clinically controlled trial of intranasal calcitonin treatment in patients with hip fracture. *Calcif Tissue Int* 2002;**71**:478–84.

Knopp JA, Diner BM, Blitz M, *et al.* Calcitonin for treating acute pain of osteoporotic vertebral compression fractures: a systematic review of randomized, controlled trials. *Osteoporos Int* 2005;**16**:1281–90.

Lyritis GP, Tsakalakos N, Magiasis B, *et al.* Analgesic effect of salmon calcitonin in osteoporotic vertebral fractures: a double blind placebo controlled study. *Calcif Tissue Int* 1991;**49**:369–72.

Tanko LB, Bagger YZ, Alexandersen P, *et al.* Safety and efficacy of a novel salmon calcitonin (sCT) technology-based oral formulation in healthy postmenopausal women: acute and 3-month effects on biomarkers of bone turnover. *J Bone Miner Res* 2004;**19**:1531-8.

Tilyard MW, Spears GFS, Thomson J, Dovey S. Treatment of postmenopausal osteoporosis with calcitriol or calcium. *N Engl J Med* 1992;**326**:357–62.

Future developments

Haguenauer D, Welch V, Shea B, *et al.* Fluoride for the treatment of postmenopausal osteoporotic fractures: a meta-analysis. *Osteoporos Int* 2000;**11**:727–38.

Kostenuik PJ. Osteoprotegerin and RANKL regulate bone resorption, density, geometry and strength. *Curr Opin Pharmacol* 2005 Sep 23; [Epub ahead of print]

LaCroix AZ, Cauley JA, Pettinger M, *et al.* Statin use, clinical fracture, and bone density in postmenopausal women: results from the Women's Health Initiative observational study. *Ann Intern Med* 2003;**139**:97–104.

Meier CR, Schlienger RG, Draenzlin ME, *et al.* HMG-CoA reductase inhibitors and risk of fractures. *JAMA* 2000;**283**:3205–10.

Mundy G, Garrett R, Harris S, *et al.* Stimulation of bone formation *in vitro* and in rodents by statins. *Science* 1999;**286**:1946–9.

Non-pharmacological interventions: calcium and vitamin D

Bischoff-Ferrari HA, Willett WC, Wong JB, *et al.* Fracture prevention with vitamin D supplementation: a meta-analysis of randomized controlled trials. *JAMA* 2005;**293**:2257–64.

Chapuy MC, Arlot ME, Duboeuf F, *et al.* Vitamin D3 and calcium to prevent hip fractures in the elderly women. *N Engl J Med* 1992;**327**:1637–42.

Grant AM, Avenell A, Campbell MK, *et al.* Oral vitamin D3 and calcium for secondary prevention of low-trauma fractures in elderly people (Randomised Evaluation of Calcium Or vitamin D, RECORD): a randomised placebo-controlled trial. *Lancet* 2005;**365**:1621–8.

Harwood RH, Sahota O, Gaynor K, *et al.* A randomised, controlled comparison of different calcium and vitamin D supplementation regimens in elderly women after hip fracture: The Nottingham Neck of Femur (NONOF) Study. *Age Ageing* 2004;**33**:45–51.

Lehtonen-Veromaa MK, Mottonen TT, *et al.* Vitamin D and attainment of peak bone mass among peripubertal Finnish girls: a 3-y prospective study. *Am J Clin Nutr* 2002;**76**:1446–53.

Nieves JW. Osteoporosis: the role of micronutrients. *Am J Clin Nutr* 2005;**81**:1232S–9S.

Porthouse J, Cockayne S, King C, *et al.* Randomised controlled trial of calcium and supplementation with cholecalciferol (vitamin D3) for prevention of fractures in primary care. *BMJ* 2005;**330**:1003–6.

Reginster JY. The high prevalence of inadequate serum vitamin D levels and implications for bone health. *Curr Med Res Opin* 2005;**21**:579–86.

Shea B, Wells G, Cranney A, Zytaruk N, *et al.* Calcium supplementation on bone loss in postmenopausal women. *Cochrane Database Syst Rev* 2004;(1):CD004526.

Trivedi DP, Doll R, Khaw KT. Effect of four monthly oral vitamin D3 (cholecalciferol) supplementation on fractures and mortality in men and women living in the community: randomised double blind controlled trial. *BMJ* 2003;**326**:469.

9 Diet, exercise and hip protectors

> Diet
> Exercise
> Hip protectors
> Further reading

Diet and regular exercise are important in protecting against cardiovascular diseases and osteoporotic fracture. Regular physical activity may also be associated with fewer vasomotor and adverse psychological symptoms. Weight-bearing and muscle-strengthening exercises contribute to maintenance of bone mass but only while they continue. Although diet and exercise modification instigated at the menopause are of benefit, it is becoming apparent that instigation much earlier – for example, in adolescence – is important to ensure that women achieve maximum benefit. Hip protectors have been introduced to provide a mechanical buffer, but evidence of patient acceptability and anti-fracture efficacy is limited.

Diet

Although the diet of many older adults is adequate, there is room for improvement for some individuals and some particular subgroups, such as those in nursing homes or long-term care. The aim is to reduce the risk of malnutrition, including obesity and undernutrition. It is becoming evident that dietary interventions should start early – even in adolescence.

Macronutrients

Macronutrients encompass fat, carbohydrate and protein. Although the healthy range of body mass index (BMI) for older adults is not established clearly, it is important that older adults consume nutrient-dense foods that are compatible with alterations in perceptions of taste and dentition with age.

Fat
Different types of fat are present in the diet, and good evidence shows that reductions in saturated fatty acids are needed to reduce the risk of coronary

heart disease (CHD). Suggestions include the use of margarine instead of butter and skimmed or semi-skimmed milk in place of full-fat milk, as well as choosing lean cuts of meat. Evidence of the benefit of long-chain omega 3 fatty acids on health, such as positive effects on cardiovascular health, insulin sensitivity and, thereby, diabetes and its associated risks, is increasing. Much of the interest in the association between omega 3 fatty acids and cardiovascular disease follows studies with Greenland Inuits who traditionally have low mortality from CHD despite a diet rich in fat. Long-chain omega 3 fatty acids can be found in oily fish.

Carbohydrate
As diets high in non-milk extrinsic sugars may displace foods that are more nutrient dense, sugars, jams, preserves and confectionery should be eaten in moderation. More emphasis is needed on other carbohydrate-rich foods (such as wholegrain breakfast cereals, grains and breads and bakery products), which would also provide fibre and a number of B vitamins. An increase in consumption of fruits and vegetables would increase intake of fibre, folate, potassium and vitamin C.

Protein
Current recommendations generally are set at the same level as for younger adults, but it is thought that this may underestimate requirements. Protein requirements are increased by illness, surgery, infection, trauma and pressure ulcers, and long-term inadequate intake of protein may result in further loss of muscle mass, impaired immune function and poor wound healing. More research is needed about the protein requirements of older adults.

Micronutrients

Micronutrients encompass vitamins and minerals. Calcium and vitamin D are covered in Chapter 8. Low intakes of a range of micronutrients, such as iron, folate and vitamin B12, can cause a number of anaemias and a range of other problems (for example, a small number of cases of reversible severe dementia have been reported in association with vitamin B12).

Antioxidants, such as selenium, vitamin E, vitamin C and beta-carotene, protect the body from damage from free radicals. Free radicals are produced during normal metabolism in the body, but they may be associated with disease and the ageing process. Several epidemiological studies have shown that people with high intakes of fruits and vegetables may have a lower risk of chronic disease than those with low intakes. The benefits of high intakes of fruits and vegetables are hypothesized to result from their antioxidant content. To date, however, no single antioxidant has been proved to prevent or decrease the risk of chronic disease, so the most practical public health advice is to increase consumption of vegetables and fruits. Supplementation with vitamin E does not prevent cancer or major cardiovascular events in healthy women and may increase the risk for heart failure in those with vascular disease or diabetes. Furthermore, a high intake of vitamin C from supplements is associated with an increased risk of mortality from cardiovascular disease in postmenopausal women with diabetes. In addition, antioxidant vitamin supplements that contain both types of vitamins do not provide cardiovascular benefit in postmenopausal women. Although one study showed that vitamin E reduced hot flushes, the difference between the active and placebo groups was not significant.

In the UK, the recommendation is to include at least five portions of fruits and vegetables per day. As the average intake for women aged 50–64 years is still less than this recommendation (3.8 portions), women should be encouraged to eat a wide variety of fruits and vegetables, as different types provide different profiles of constituents.

In 2003, the Food Standards Agency's Expert Committee on Vitamins and Minerals in the UK set safe upper limits for some vitamins and minerals, including several of the antioxidant nutrients (Table 9.1). Vitamin and mineral supplements may be beneficial to some subgroups of the population, but evidence shows that excessive intakes of some vitamins and minerals can cause harm.

Table 9.1

Safe upper levels for intake of selected antioxidants. Source: Expert Group on Vitamins and Minerals, Food Standards Agency (2003)

Nutrient	Safe upper level (per day)
Beta-carotene	9 mg
Selenium	0.45 mg
Vitamin E	800 IU (540 mg d-α-tocopherol equivalents/day)
Vitamin C	Insufficient evidence

Functional foods

Functional foods are generally defined as foods that confer a 'benefit' to the host beyond simple nutrition. Five main types of functional foods show promise in women's health:

- probiotics
- prebiotics
- synbiotics
- nutraceuticals
- fibre.

Probiotics

A probiotic is defined as a 'live microbial feed supplement which beneficially affects the host animal by improving its intestinal balance'. Currently, the best studied probiotics are the lactic acid bacteria, particularly *Lactobacillus* spp. and *Bifidobacterium* spp. These can be combined with food products such as cereals, bioyoghurts and drinks. Increasing evidence shows the potential of probiotics in benefiting gastrointestinal conditions (such as diarrhoea and irritable bowel syndrome) and non-gastrointestinal tract conditions (such as candidiasis and urinary tract and respiratory tract infections).

Prebiotics

Prebiotics are 'non-digestible food ingredients which selectively stimulate a limited number of bacteria in the colon, to improve host health'. The emphasis of prebiotic research, therefore, is to enhance the indigenous probiotic flora. This includes strategies to develop specific prebiotics for individual probiotic organisms, as well as aiding persistence of prebiotic effects throughout the gastrointestinal tract. They may be involved in calcium absorption.

Synbiotics

Synbiotics contain complementary probiotic and prebiotic ingredients that interact to provide a synergistic effect towards the maintenance of a desirable microbial population in the intestinal microbiota. This is a developing area of functional foods, and few clinical studies of their impact on human health have been performed to date.

Nutraceuticals

Nutraceuticals are natural components of foods (such as isoflavones and phytoestrogens) that may be released during digestion and therefore become bioavailable. These are discussed in Chapter 10. Such compounds may have a direct health effect on the host or an indirect health effect via the microflora, or both.

Fibre

Dietary fibre consists of plant substances that resist hydrolysis by digestive enzymes in the small bowel and is an extremely complex group of substances. Fibre can be classified according to its solubility and fermentability by bacteria: a soluble fibre is readily fermentable by colonic bacteria and an insoluble fibre is only slowly fermentable. Fibres may act in several ways, including through gel-forming effects in the stomach and small intestine, fermentation by colonic bacteria, a 'mop and sponge' effect and concomitant changes in other aspects of the diet. These actions lead to potentially beneficial effects both in the gastrointestinal tract and systemically, such as lowering levels of cholesterol in serum and improving glycaemic control.

The Mediterranean diet

The Mediterranean diet is characterized by a high intake of vegetables, legumes, fruits and cereals (in the past largely unrefined); a moderate to high intake of fish; a low intake of saturated lipids but a high intake of unsaturated lipids, particularly olive oil; a low to moderate intake of dairy products, mostly cheese and yogurt; a low intake of meat; and a modest intake of ethanol, mostly as wine. Several studies have found associations between Mediterranean and modified Mediterranean diets and reductions in mortality. The benefit of a Mediterranean type diet does not seem to be limited to Mediterranean countries and has been found in other countries, such as Australia.

Exercise

A large body of research has established that regular physical activity for postmenopausal women reduces the risk of osteoporotic fractures, CHD and type 2 diabetes mellitus. Furthermore, hot flushes, urinary incontinence, insomnia and depression may also be improved by physical activity. Exercise methods can be divided into three general categories:

- endurance exercise (aerobic)
- strength exercise (resistance)
- balance exercises (such as Tai Chi).

Exercise and osteoporosis

The role of exercise in preventing osteoporotic fractures is well established; however, what type, intensity, frequency and duration of activity are most effective is unclear. A Cochrane review assessed the influence on bone mineral density (BMD) of different exercise regimens two to three times a week over 12 months in menopausal women. Fast walking effectively improved bone density in the spine and the hip, whereas, on available evidence, weight-bearing exercises were associated with increases in bone density of the spine but not the hip. Exercise regimens can be very helpful in the management of established osteoporosis. The benefits are mainly related to increased wellbeing, muscle strength, postural stability and a reduction of chronic pain rather than an increase of skeletal mass. Exercise has to be structured carefully, because of concerns about falls and fractures.

Exercise and coronary heart disease

Exercise has a direct effect on the cardiovascular system by increasing oxygen delivery and utilization and by decreasing the risk of ventricular arrhythmias and the overall risk of sudden cardiac death. In addition, physical activity can increase levels of high-density lipoprotein cholesterol. The indirect effects of exercise in modifying risk factors for CHD, such as reductions in body weight, may be the most important factor in diminishing risk. Exercise may also prevent progression of atherosclerosis. Again, the optimal type, frequency and intensity are uncertain. Low-intensity exercise, such as walking (with which fewer concerns about falls exist), can reduce the risk of cardiovascular disease to a degree similar to that achieved with more vigorous physical activity.

Exercise and urinary incontinence

Pelvic floor exercises are used commonly for stress incontinence. They are also used in the treatment of women with mixed incontinence, and less commonly for urge incontinence. Adjuncts, such as biofeedback or electrical stimulation, are also commonly used with training of the muscle of the pelvic floor. The content of programmes for training of the muscle of the pelvic floor is highly variable. Systematic review has found that training of the muscle of the pelvic floor seemed to be an effective treatment for adult women with stress or mixed incontinence and better than no treatment or placebo treatments. The role of training of the pelvic floor muscle for women with urge incontinence alone remains unclear. Most data were obtained in premenopausal rather than postmenopausal women, and further studies are awaited.

Hip protectors

These are used to reduce the impact of falling directly on the hip. Hip protectors (Figure 9.1) are not particularly attractive, however, and are uncomfortable in hot weather, as well as being difficult to fit easily. Systematic review has found no evidence of effectiveness of hip protectors from studies in which randomization was by individual patients within an institution or for those living in their own homes. Data from randomized cluster studies indicate that, for those who live in institutional care with a high background incidence of hip fracture, a programme in which hip protectors are provided seems to reduce the incidence of hip fractures. A randomized controlled trial of women older than 70 years at high risk of hip fracture who lived in the community in the UK found no benefit.

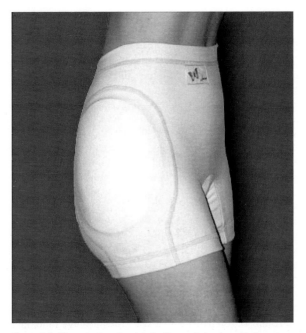

Figure 9.1 Hip protectors. Reprinted with permission from HipSaver Inc., Canton, MA, USA

Further reading

Diet

Chenoy R, Hussain S, Tayob Y, *et al*. Effect of oral gamolenic acid from evening primrose oil on menopausal flushing. *BMJ* 1994;**308**:501–3.

Chicago Dietetic Association, South Suburban Dietetic Association and Dietitians of Canada. *Manual of Clinical Dietetics*. Chicago: American Dietetic Association, 2000.

de Vrese M, Schrezenmeir J. Probiotics and non-intestinal infectious conditions. *Br J Nutr* 2002; **88**(Suppl 1):S59–66.

Din JN, Newby DE, Flapan AD. Omega 3 fatty acids and cardiovascular disease – fishing for a natural treatment. *BMJ* 2004;**328**:30–5.

Food Standards Agency, Expert Group on Vitamins and Minerals. *Safe Upper Levels for Vitamins and Minerals*. London: Food Standards Agency, 2003. Available at: http://www.food.gov.uk/ (last accessed 29 September 2005).

Frazier AL, Li L, Cho E, *et al*. Adolescent diet and risk of breast cancer. *Cancer Causes Control* 2004;**15**:73–82.

James SL, Muir JG, Curtis SL, Gibson PR. Dietary fibre: a roughage guide. *Intern Med J* 2003;**33**:291–6.

Kennedy E, Meyers L. Dietary Reference Intakes: development and uses for assessment of micronutrient status of women – a global perspective. *Am J Clin Nutr* 2005;**81**:1194S–7S.

Knoops KT, de Groot LC, Kromhout D, *et al.* Mediterranean diet, lifestyle factors, and 10-year mortality in elderly European men and women: the HALE project. *JAMA* 2004;**292**:1433–9.

Kouris-Blazos A, Gnardellis C, Wahlqvist ML, *et al.* Are the advantages of the Mediterranean diet transferable to other populations? A cohort study in Melbourne, Australia. *Br J Nutr* 1999;**82**:57–61.

La Vecchia C. Mediterranean diet and cancer. *Public Health Nutr* 2004;**7**:965-8.

Lee DH, Folsom AR, Harnack L, *et al.* Does supplemental vitamin C increase cardiovascular disease risk in women with diabetes? *Am J Clin Nutr* 2004;**80**:1194–200.

Lee IM, Cook NR, Gaziano JM, *et al.* Vitamin E in the primary prevention of cardiovascular disease and cancer: the Women's Health Study: a randomized controlled trial. *JAMA* 2005;**294**:56–65.

Lonn E, Bosch J, Yusuf S, *et al.* Effects of long-term vitamin E supplementation on cardiovascular events and cancer. a randomized controlled trial. *JAMA* 2005;**293**:1338–47.

McKevith B. Role of diet. In: Rees M, Mander T, eds. *Managing the Menopause without Oestrogen*. London: RSM Press, 2004:69–73.

Millward DJ, Jackson AA. Protein/energy ratios of current diets in developed and developing countries compared with a safe protein/energy ratio: implications for recommended protein and amino acid intakes. *Public Health Nutr* 2004;**7**:387–405.

Smejkal C. Functional foods. In: Rees M, Mander T, eds. *Managing the Menopause without Oestrogen*. London: RSM Press, 2004:75–9.

Trichopoulou A, Orfanos P, Norat T, *et al.* Modified Mediterranean diet and survival: EPIC-elderly prospective cohort study. *BMJ* 2005;**330**:991.

Waters DD, Alderman EL, Hsia J, *et al.* Effects of hormone replacement therapy and antioxidant vitamin supplements on coronary atherosclerosis in postmenopausal women: a randomized controlled trial. *JAMA* 2002;**288**:2432–40.

Wright JD, Wang C-Y, Kennedy-Stephenson J, *et al. Dietary Intake of Ten Key Nutrients for Public Health, United States: 1999–2000. Advance Data from Vital and Health Statistics; No. 334.* Hyattsville, MD: National Center for Health Statistics, 2003.

Exercise and hip protectors

Aiello EJ, Yasui Y, Tworoger SS, *et al.* Effect of a yearlong, moderate-intensity exercise intervention on the occurrence and severity of menopause symptoms in postmenopausal women. *Menopause* 2004;**11**:382–8.

Asikainen TM, Kukkonen-Harjula K, Miilunpalo S. Exercise for health for early postmenopausal women: a systematic review of randomised controlled trials. *Sports Med* 2004;**34**:753–78.

Birks YF, Porthouse J, Addie C, *et al.* Randomized controlled trial of hip protectors among women living in the community. *Osteoporos Int* 2004;**15**:701–6.

Bonaiuti D, Shea B, Iovine R, *et al.* Exercise for preventing and treating osteoporosis in postmenopausal women. *Cochrane Database Syst Rev* 2003;(**4**):CD0000333.

Hay-Smith EJ, Bo Berghmans LC, Hendriks HJ, *et al.* Pelvic floor muscle training for urinary incontinence in women. *Cochrane Database Syst Rev* 2001;(1):CD001407.

Lindh-Astrand L, Nedstrand E, Wyon Y, Hammar M. Vasomotor symptoms and quality of life in previously sedentary postmenopausal women randomised to physical activity or estrogen therapy. *Maturitas* 2004;48:97–105.

Manson JE, Greenland P, LaCroix AZ, *et al.* Walking compared with vigorous exercise for the prevention of cardiovascular events in women. *N Engl J Med* 2002; 347:716–25.

Oehler MK. Exercise and physical interventions. In: Rees M, Mander T, eds. *Managing the Menopause without Oestrogen.* London: RSM Press, 2004:81–5.

Parker MJ, Gillespie LD, Gillespie WJ. Hip protectors for preventing hip fractures in the elderly. *Cochrane Database Syst Rev* 2004;(3):CD001255.

Qin L, Choy W, Leung K, *et al.* Beneficial effects of regular Tai Chi exercise on musculoskeletal system. *J Bone Miner Metab* 2005;23:186–90.

Uusi-Rasi K, Sievanen H, Heinonen A, *et al.* Determinants of changes in bone mass and femoral neck structure, and physical performance after menopause: a 9-year follow-up of initially peri-menopausal women. *Osteoporos Int* 2005;16:616–22.

Vainionpaa A, Korpelainen R, Leppaluoto J, Jamsa T. Effects of high-impact exercise on bone mineral density: a randomized controlled trial in premenopausal women. *Osteoporos Int* 2005;16:191–7.

Wildman RP, Schott LL, Brockwell S, *et al.* A dietary and exercise intervention slows menopause-associated progression of subclinical atherosclerosis as measured by intima-media thickness of the carotid arteries. *J Am Coll Cardiol* 2004;44:579–85.

10 Alternative and complementary therapies

Phytoestrogens
Herbalism
Homeopathy
Dehydroepiandrosterone (DHEA)
Progesterone transdermal creams
Mechanical
Further reading

Evidence from randomized trials that alternative and complementary therapies improve menopausal symptoms or have the same benefits as hormone replacement therapy (HRT) is poor. Many women, however, use them in the belief that they are safer and 'more natural', especially with the concerns about the safety of oestrogen-based HRT after publication of the Women's Health Initiative study and Million Women Study. In the UK, more than one in 10 adults visit a therapist each year, and nearly half are taking an over-the-counter food supplement. Similar figures are available in the US. The choice is confusing. A major concern is interaction with other treatments with potentially fatal consequences. Some herbal preparations may contain oestrogenic compounds, and this is a concern for women with hormone-dependent diseases, such as breast cancer. Concern also exists about the quality control of production.

Phytoestrogens

Phytoestrogens are plant substances that have effects similar to those of oestrogens. Preparations vary from enriched foods, such as bread or drinks (soy milk), to more concentrated tablets. The most important groups are called isoflavones and lignans. The major isoflavones are genistein and daidzein. The major lignans are enterolactone and enterodiol.

Isoflavones are found in soybeans, chickpeas, red clover and probably other legumes (beans and peas). Oilseeds such as flaxseed are rich in lignans, and they are also found in cereal bran, whole cereals, vegetables, legumes and fruit.

The role of phytoestrogens has stimulated considerable interest, as people from populations that consume a diet high in isoflavones, such as the

Japanese, seem to have lower rates of menopausal vasomotor symptoms; cardiovascular disease; osteoporosis; and breast, colon, endometrial and ovarian cancers. With regard to menopausal symptoms, the evidence from randomized placebo-controlled trials in Western populations is conflicting for soy and derivatives of red clover. Similarly, debate also surrounds the effects on lipoproteins, endothelial function, blood pressure, cognition and the endometrium. The isoflavone daidzein is metabolized extensively in the gut to the more oestrogenic secondary metabolite equol by the human gut microflora. That only 30% of Western populations excrete high levels of equol might account for the conflicting evidence provided by clinical trials.

Phytoestrogens and the synthetic isoflavone ipriflavone may maintain bone mass, but the evidence is conflicting. Phytoestrogens exert biphasic dose-dependent effects on osteoblasts and osteoprogenitor cells, stimulating osteogenesis at low concentrations and inhibiting osteogenesis at high concentrations. They inhibit osteoclast formation and activity. Some short-term studies suggest a beneficial effect, but the optimal dose is as yet unknown. Studies are underway, including a European Union Study (Phytos), which may help resolve these issues. Of concern, ipriflavone may induce lymphocytopenia in a significant number of women.

Further well-designed, randomized trials are needed to determine the role and safety of phytoestrogen supplements in perimenopausal and postmenopausal women.

Herbalism

Herbal remedies need to be used with caution in women with a contraindication to oestrogen, as some herbs – for example, ginseng – have oestrogenic properties (Box 10.1). The consequences of herb–drug interactions include bleeding when combined with warfarin or aspirin; hypertension, coma and mild serotonin syndrome when combined with serotonin reuptake inhibitors; and reduced efficacy of antiepileptics and oral contraceptives. For example, *ginkgo biloba* (ginkgo) can cause bleeding when combined with warfarin or aspirin, high blood pressure when combined with a thiazide diuretic and even coma when combined with trazodone. *Panax ginseng* (ginseng) reduces the blood concentrations of alcohol and warfarin and can induce mania when used concomitantly with phenelzine. *Hypericum perforatum* (St John's wort) reduces the blood concentrations of cyclosporin, midazolam, tacrolimus, amitriptyline, digoxin, warfarin and theophylline. Cases have been reported in which reduced concentrations of cyclosporin have led to organ rejection. *Hypericum* also causes breakthrough bleeding and unplanned pregnancies when used concomitantly with oral contraceptives. It also causes serotonin syndrome when used in combination with selective

---

Box 10.1

Herbs used by menopausal women

Actaea racemosa (*black cohosh*)
Piper methysticum (*kava kava*)
Oenothera bienis (*evening primrose*)
Angelica sinensis (*dong quai*)
Ginkgo biloba (*gingko*)
Panax ginseng (*ginseng*)
Others, such as wild yam cream, St John's wort, *Agnus castus* (Chasteberry), liquorice root and *Valerian* root

---

serotonin reuptake inhibitors (for example, sertraline and paroxetine). Furthermore, little control over the quality of the products exists, so it is unusual to know what is actually present in individual herbal preparations and dietary supplements. Severe adverse reactions, including renal and liver failure and cancer, have been reported. Moreover, some preparations contain high levels of heavy metals, such as arsenic, lead and mercury. The safety of some herbs, such as kava kava, has been questioned. Worldwide regulatory supervision of herbal medicines – and the claims made for them – is required.

Actaea racemosa (black cohosh)

Actaea racemosa (formerly known as *Cimicifuga racemosa*), a herbaceous perennial plant native to North America, is used widely to alleviate menopausal symptoms. Early animal studies suggest an 'oestrogen-like' activity; more recent work suggests the effects may result from a central activity.

The results from placebo-controlled trials or comparison with conjugated equine oestrogens are promising, but little is known about the long-term safety and toxicity.

Piper methysticum (kava kava)

In the South Pacific, kava kava has been used for recreational and medicinal purposes for thousands of years. A Cochrane review concluded that it may be an effective symptomatic treatment for anxiety, but the data about menopausal symptoms are conflicting. Concern about liver damage has led regulatory authorities to suspend or withdraw kava kava.

Oenothera biennis (evening primrose)

Evening primrose oil is rich in gamma-linolenic acid. One small, placebo-controlled, randomized trial showed it to be ineffective for treating hot flushes.

Angelica sinensis (dong quai)

Dong quai is a perennial plant native to southwest China that is used commonly in traditional Chinese medicine. It was not found to be superior to placebo in a randomized trial. Interaction with warfarin and photosensitization have been reported.

Ginkgo biloba (gingko)

The use of *Gingko biloba* is widespread, but little evidence shows that it improves menopausal symptoms.

Panax ginseng (ginseng)

Ginseng is a perennial herb native to Korea and China and has been used extensively in eastern Asia. It was not found to be superior to placebo in a randomized trial. Case reports have associated ginseng with postmenopausal bleeding and mastalgia. Interactions have been observed with warfarin, phenelzine and alcohol.

Other herbs

Wild yam cream, St John's wort, *Agnus castus* (Chasteberry), liquorice root and *Valerian* root are also popular, but no good evidence shows that they have any effect on menopausal symptoms. Claims have been made that steroids (diosgenein) in yams (dioscorea villosa) can be converted in the body to progesterone, but this is biochemically impossible in humans.

Homeopathy

Samuel Hahnemann (1755–1843), a German physician and scientist, was the first to enunciate the central tenets of homeopathic philosophy. He believed in a 'vital force' that animates and regulates the human form and directs growth, healing and repair. He postulated that the homoeopathic remedy acted through the vital force, stimulating a healing or self-regulating response. He then put forward the principle of 'similars', which claims that patients with particular signs and symptoms can be cured if given a drug that produces the same signs and symptoms in a healthy individual. He then pursued the concept of minimum dose – the smallest amount of a substance that could be given to avoid side-effects and yet would still bring about a healing response. He found that the curative action of certain preparations seemed to be stronger at some of the lower doses, particularly when shaken vigorously (a process known as succession), than at higher doses. The mechanisms that underlie the biological response to ultramolecular dilutions, however, are scientifically unclear. Data from case histories, observational studies and a small number of randomized trials are encouraging, but more research clearly is needed.

Dehydroepiandrosterone

Dehydroepiandrosterone (DHEA) is a steroid secreted by the adrenal cortex. It is mostly produced in a sulphated form (DHEA-S), which may be converted to DHEA in many tissues. Blood levels of DHEA decrease dramatically with age. This led to suggestions that the effects of ageing can be counteracted by DHEA 'replacement therapy'. Dehydroepiandrosterone is increasingly being used in the US, where it is classed as a food supplement, for its supposed anti-ageing effects. Some studies have shown benefits on the skeleton, cognition, wellbeing, libido and the vagina. No evidence shows that DHEA has any effect on hot flushes. The short-term effects of taking DHEA are still controversial, and possible harmful effects of long-term use are as yet unknown.

Progesterone transdermal creams

Progesterone has been prepared in gels and creams for a number of years. One licensed gel is available in Europe; however, it is indicated for local use on the breast but not for systemic therapy. A vaginal gel for endometrial protection has been studied.

The various transdermal preparations for systemic use usually contain micronized progesterone in concentrations ranging from 0.17 mg/g to 64.0 mg/g, with most products containing about 30.0 mg/g in a cream. Progesterone creams have been advocated for the treatment of menopausal symptoms and skeletal protection. At present, there are insufficient published data to show if transdermal progesterone has a positive effect on vasomotor symptoms or the skeleton. To avoid side-effects of progestogens, women who take systemic oestrogens may use transdermal progesterone creams for endometrial protection. No consistent evidence, however, shows that transdermal progesterone creams can prevent mitotic activity or induce secretory change in an oestrogen-primed endometrium. Thus, women who use such a combination are increasing their risk of endometrial cancer, and the practice should be discouraged. Further research is needed to establish whether progesterone creams have any role to play in the management of the short- and long-term consequences of the menopause.

'Mechanical'

The term 'mechanical' is used, as these therapies do not involve ingestion or application of any agent. These include acupuncture, reflexology, acupressure, Alexander technique, Ayurveda, osteopathy and Reiki. These have been covered in recent reviews and need further examination in relation to the menopause.

Acupuncture

Acupuncture is the stimulation of special points on the body, usually by the insertion of fine needles, and originated in the Far East about 2000 years ago (Figure 10.1). In its original form, acupuncture was based on the principles of traditional Chinese medicine. According to these, the workings of the human body are controlled by a vital force or energy called 'Qi' (pronounced 'chee'), which circulates between the organs along channels called meridians. There are 12 main meridians, and these correspond to 12 major functions or 'organs' of the body. Qi energy must flow in the correct strength and quality through each of these meridians and organs for health to be maintained. The acupuncture points are located along the meridians and provide one means of altering the flow of Qi. A randomized controlled trial of electro-acupuncture showed no benefit for menopausal symptoms.

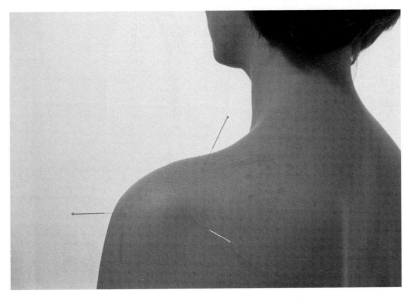

Figure 10.1 Acupuncture needles. Courtesy of British Acupuncture Council

Reflexology

Reflexology aims to relieve stress or treat health conditions through the application of pressure to specific points or areas of the feet. The underlying idea of reflexology is that areas of the feet correspond to (and affect) other parts of the body (Figure 10.2). In some cases, pressure may also be applied to the hands or ears. Techniques similar to reflexology have been used for thousands of years in Egypt, China and other areas. Although it has been used for various conditions such as pain, anxiety and premenstrual syndrome, few studies have looked at menopausal complaints. One randomized trial has been published so far, and no improvement of vasomotor symptoms was found. Currently, its use is thus uncertain.

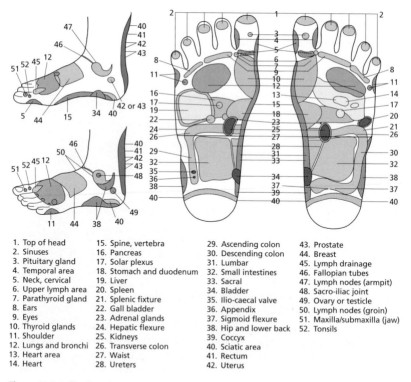

1. Top of head
2. Sinuses
3. Pituitary gland
4. Temporal area
5. Neck, cervical
6. Upper lymph area
7. Parathyroid gland
8. Ears
9. Eyes
10. Thyroid glands
11. Shoulder
12. Lungs and bronchi
13. Heart area
14. Heart

15. Spine, vertebra
16. Pancreas
17. Solar plexus
18. Stomach and duodenum
19. Liver
20. Spleen
21. Splenic fixture
22. Gall bladder
23. Adrenal glands
24. Hepatic flexure
25. Kidneys
26. Transverse colon
27. Waist
28. Ureters

29. Ascending colon
30. Descending colon
31. Lumbar
32. Small intestines
33. Sacral
34. Bladder
35. Ilio-caecal valve
36. Appendix
37. Sigmoid flexure
38. Hip and lower back
39. Coccyx
40. Sciatic area
41. Rectum
42. Uterus

43. Prostate
44. Breast
45. Lymph drainage
46. Fallopian tubes
47. Lymph nodes (armpit)
48. Sacro-iliac joint
49. Ovary or testicle
50. Lymph nodes (groin)
51. Maxilla/submaxilla (jaw)
52. Tonsils

Figure 10.2 Reflexology chart

Further reading

General

Ernst E, Pittler MH, Stevinson C, White AR. *The Desktop Guide to Complementary and Alternative Medicine.* Edinburgh: Mosby, 2001.

Gokhale L, Sturdee DW, Parsons AD. The use of food supplements among women attending menopause clinics in the West Midlands. *J Br Menopause Soc* 2003;**9**:32–5.

Kam IW, Dennehy CE, Tsourounis C. Dietary supplement use among menopausal women attending a San Francisco health conference. *Menopause* 2002;**9**:72–8.

Myers SP, Cheras PA. The other side of the coin: safety of complementary and alternative medicine. *Med J Aust* 2004;**181**:222–5.

Saper RB, Kales SN, Paquin J, *et al.* Heavy metal content of ayurvedic herbal medicine products. *JAMA* 2004;**292**:2868–73.

Thomas KJ, Nicholl JP, Coleman P. Use and expenditure on complementary medicine in England: a population based survey. *Complement Ther Med* 2001;**9**:2–11.

Websites

National Center for Complementary and Alternative Medicine. *Alternative therapies for managing menopausal symptoms* http://nccam.nih.gov/health/alerts/ menopause

National Institutes for Health Office of Dietary Supplements http://dietary-supplements.info.nih.gov

Office of Dietary Supplements. IBIDS database http://ods.od.nih.gov/databases/ibids.html

Phytoestrogens

Atkinson C, Compston JE, Day NE, *et al.* The effects of phytoestrogen isoflavones on bone density in women: a double-blind, randomized, placebo-controlled trial. *Am J Clin Nutr* 2004;**79**:326–33.

Alexandersen P, Toussaint A, Christiansen C, *et al.* Ipriflavone in the treatment of postmenopausal osteoporosis. *JAMA* 2001;**285**:1482–8.

Branca F. Dietary phyto-oestrogens and bone health. *Proc Nutr Soc* 2003;**62**:877-87.

Crisafulli A, Marini H, Bitto A, *et al.* Effects of genistein on hot flushes in early postmenopausal women: a randomized, double-blind EPT- and placebo-controlled study. *Menopause* 2004;**11**:400–4.

Dang ZC, Lowik C. Dose-dependent effects of phytoestrogens on bone. *Trends Endocrinol Metab* 2005;**16**:207–13.

Dodin S, Lemay A, Jacques H, *et al.* The effects of flaxseed dietary supplement on lipid profile, bone mineral density, and symptoms in menopausal women: a randomized, double-blind, wheat germ placebo-controlled clinical trial. *J Clin Endocrinol Metab* 2005;**90**:1390–7.

Faure ED, Chantre P, Mares P. Effects of a standardized soy extract on hot flushes: a multicenter, double-blind, randomized, placebo-controlled study. *Menopause* 2002;**9**:329–34.

Kreijkamp-Kaspers S, Kok L, Grobbee DE, *et al*. Effect of soy protein containing isoflavones on cognitive function, bone mineral density, and plasma lipids in postmenopausal women: a randomized controlled trial. *JAMA* 2004;292:65–74.

Krebs EE, Ensrud KE, MacDonald R, Wilt TJ. Phytoestrogens for treatment of menopausal symptoms: a systematic review. *Obstet Gynecol* 2004;104:824–36.

Penotti M, Fabio E, Modena AB, *et al*. Effect of soy-derived isoflavones on hot flushes, endometrial thickness, and the pulsatility index of the uterine and cerebral arteries. *Fertil Steril* 2003;79:1112–17.

Rowland IR, Wiseman H, Sanders TA, *et al*. Interindividual variation in metabolism of soy isoflavones and lignans: influence of habitual diet on equol production by the gut microflora. *Nutr Cancer* 2000;36:27–32.

Schult TM, Ensrud KE, Blackwell T, *et al*. Effect of isoflavones on lipids and bone turnover markers in menopausal women. *Maturitas* 2004;48:209–18.

Tice JA, Ettinger B, Ensrud K, *et al*. Phytoestrogen supplements for the treatment of hot flashes: the Isoflavone Clover Extract (ICE) Study: a randomized controlled trial. *JAMA* 2003;290:207–14.

Unfer V, Casini ML, Costabile L, *et al*. Endometrial effects of long-term treatment with phytoestrogens: a randomized, double-blind, placebo-controlled study. *Fertil Steril* 2004;82:145–8.

Van de Weijer PHM, Barentsen R. Isoflavones from red clover (Promensil®) significantly reduce menopausal hot flush symptoms compared with placebo. *Maturitas* 2002;42:187–93.

Herbalism

Boon H, Smith M. *The botanical pharmacy*. Ontario: Quarry Press Inc, 1999.

Borrelli F, Izzo AA, Ernst E. Pharmacological effects of *Cimicifuga racemosa*. *Life Sci* 2003;73:1215–29.

Cagnacci A, Arangino S, Renzi A, *et al*. Kava-kava administration reduces anxiety in perimenopausal women. *Maturitas* 2003;44:103–9.

Dailey RK, Neale AV, Northrup J, *et al*. Herbal product use and menopause symptom relief in primary care patients: a MetroNet study. *J Womens Health* 2003;12:633–41.

Davis SR, Briganti EM, Chen RQ, *et al*. The effects of Chinese medicinal herbs on postvasomotor symptoms of Australian women. *Med J Aust* 2001;174:68–71.

Garvey GJ, Hahn G, Lee RV, Harbison RD. Heavy metal hazards of Asian traditional remedies. *Int J Environ Health Res* 2001;11:63–71.

Grube B, Walper A, Wheatley D. St John's wort extract: efficacy for menopausal symptoms of psychological origin. *Adv Ther* 1999;16:177–86.

Hartley DE, Heinze L, Elsabagh S, File SE. Effects on cognition and mood in postmenopausal women of 1-week treatment with *Ginkgo biloba*. *Pharmacol Biochem Behaviour* 2003;75:711–20.

Hernandez Munoz G, Pluchino S. *Cimicifuga racemosa* for the treatment of hot flushes in women surviving breast cancer. *Maturitas* 2003;44(Suppl 1):S59–65.

Hirata JD, Small R, Swiersz LM, *et al*. Does dong quai have estrogenic effects in postmenopausal women? A double-blind, placebo controlled trial. *Fertil Steril* 1997;68:981–7.

Hu Z, Yang X, Ho PC, *et al.* Herb-drug interactions: a literature review. *Drugs* 2005;**65**:1239–82.

Hudson TS, Standish L, Breed C, *et al.* Clinical and endocrinological effects of a menopausal botanical formula. *J Naturopath Med* 1999;**7**:73–7.

Huntley A, Ernst E. A systematic review of the safety of black cohosh. *Menopause* 2003;**10**:58–64.

Komesaroff PA, Black CVS, Cable V, Sudhir K. Effects of wild yam extract on menopausal symptoms, lipids and sex hormones in healthy menopausal women. *Climacteric* 2001;**4**:144–50.

Kraft M, Spahn TW, Menzel J, *et al.* Fulminant liver failure after administration of the herbal antidepressant Kava-Kava. *Dtsch Med Wochenschr* 2001;**126**:970–2.

Laino C. *Black Cohosh linked to Autoimmune Hepatitis.* New York: Medscape, 2003. Available at: http://www.medscape.com/viewarticle/463059 (last accessed 6th October 2005).

Nortier JL, Martinez MC, Schmeiser HH, *et al.* Urothelial carcinoma associated with the use of a chinese herb (*Aristolochia fangchi*). *N Engl J Med* 2000;**342**:1686–92.

Pittler MH, Ernst E. Kava extract for treating anxiety. *Cochrane Database Syst Rev* 2003;(4):CD003383.

Thompson Coon J, Ernst E. Panax ginseng: a systematic review of adverse effects and drug interactions. *Drug Saf* 2002;**25**:323–44.

Whiting PW, Clouston A, Kerlin P. Black cohosh and other herbal remedies associated with acute hepatitis. *Med J Aust* 2002;**177**:432–5.

Wiklund IK, Mattsson LA, Lindgren R, *et al.* Effects of a standardised ginseng extract on quality of life and physiological parameters in symptomatic postmenopausal women: a double blind, placebo controlled trial. *Int J Clin Pharmacol Res* 1999;**9**:89–99.

Wuttke W, Seidlova-Wuttke D, Gorkow C. The *Cimicifuga* preparation BNO 1055 vs. conjugated estrogens in a double blind placebo-controlled study: effects on menopause symptoms and bone markers. *Maturitas* 2003;**44**(Suppl 1):S67–77.

Homeopathy

Clover A, Ratsey D. Homeopathic treatment of hot flushes: a pilot study. *Homeopathy* 2002;**91**:75–9.

Jacobs J, Herman P, Heron K, *et al.* Homeopathy for menopausal symptoms in breast cancer survivors: a preliminary randomized controlled trial. *J Altern Complement Med* 2005;**11**:21–7.

Thompson EA. Homeopathy and the menopause. *J Br Menopause Soc* 2002;**8**:151–4.

Thompson EA, Montgomery A, Douglas D, Reilly D. A pilot, randomized, double-blinded, placebo-controlled trial of individualized homeopathy for symptoms of estrogen withdrawal in breast-cancer survivors. *J Altern Complement Med* 2005;**11**:13–20.

Dehydroepiandrosterone

Hirshman E, Wells E, Wierman ME, *et al.* The effect of dehydroepiandrosterone (DHEA) on recognition memory decision processes and discrimination in postmenopausal women. *Psychon Bull Rev* 2003;**10**:125–34.

Lasley BL, Santoro N, Randolf JF, *et al.* Metabolic effects of dehydroepiandrosterone testosterone, and estradiol to stages of the menopausal transition and ethnicity. *J Clin Endocrinol Metab* 2002;**87**:3760–7.

Lasco A, Frisina N, Morabito N, *et al.* The relationship of circulating replacement therapy in postmenopausal women. *Eur J Endocrinol* 2001;**145**:457–61.

Marcelli C. Can DHEA be used to prevent bone loss and osteoporosis? *Joint Bone Spine* 2003;**70**:1–2.

Progesterone transdermal creams

Leonetti H, Longo S, Ansti JN. Transdermal progesterone cream for vasomotor symptoms and postmenopausal bone loss. *Obstet Gynecol* 1999;**94**:225–8.

Lydeking-Olsen E, Beck-Jensen JE, Setchell KD, Holm-Jensen T. Soymilk or progesterone for prevention of bone loss – a 2 year randomized, placebo-controlled trial. *Eur J Nutr* 2004;**43**:246–57.

Wren BG. Transdermal progesterone creams for postmenopausal women: more hype than hope? *Med J Aust* 2005;**182**:237–9.

Wren BG, Champion SM, Willetts K, *et al.* Transdermal progesterone and its effect on vasomotor symptoms, blood lipid levels, bone metabolic markers, moods, and quality of life for postmenopausal women. *Menopause* 2003;**10**:13–18.

'Mechanical'

Ernst E. Clinical effectiveness of acupuncture: an overview of systematic reviews. In: Ernst E, White A, eds. *Acupuncture, A Scientific Appraisal.* Oxford: Butterworth Heinemann, 1999:107–27.

Ernst E, Köder K. An overview of reflexology. *Eur J Gen Pract* 1997;**3**:52–7.

Sandberg M, Wijma K, Wyon Y, Nedstrand E, Hammar M. Effects of electro-acupuncture on psychological distress in postmenopausal women. *Complement Ther Med* 2002;**10**:161–9.

Williamson J, White A, Hart A, Ernst E. Randomised controlled trial of reflexology for menopausal symptoms. *BJOG* 2002;**109**:1050–5.

WOMEN WITH SPECIAL NEEDS

11 Premature menopause

Introduction

Ideally, premature menopause should be defined as menopause that occurs at an age more than two standard deviations below the mean estimated for the reference population. In the absence of reliable estimates of age of natural menopause in developing countries, the age of 40 years is used frequently as an arbitrary limit below which the menopause is said to be premature. In the developed world, however, the age of 45 years should be taken as the cut-off point.

The condition is not uncommon. Overall, premature ovarian failure (POF) is responsible for 4–18% of cases of secondary amenorrhoea and 10–28% of primary amenorrhoea. It is estimated to affect 1% of women younger than 40 years and 0.1% of those under 30 years.

Aetiology

Primary premature ovarian failure

Primary POF can occur at any age, even in children. It can present as primary or secondary amenorrhoea. In the great majority of cases, no cause can be found. Although these women are generally considered to be infertile, spontaneous ovarian activity may occur with the resulting implications of fertility and pregnancy. Traditional texts have concentrated on describing ovarian failure as being associated with a deficient number of primordial follicles from the onset of menarche, accelerated follicle atresia or follicles resistant to stimulation by gonadotrophins. In the absence of a non-invasive test to differentiate between follicular depletion or dysfunction, the only

---

Box 11.1

Causes of premature ovarian failure

Primary
Chromosome abnormalities
Follicle-stimulating hormone receptor gene polymorphism and inhibin B
  mutation
Enzyme deficiencies
Autoimmune disease

Secondary
Chemotherapy and radiotherapy
Bilateral oophorectomy or surgical menopause
Hysterectomy without oophorectomy
Infection

---

alternative is laparoscopic ovarian biopsy. The validity of single biopsies has been questioned, with pregnancies occurring despite histological lack of follicles in the biopsy material.

The causes are detailed in Box 11.1.

Chromosome abnormalities

The requirement for two intact X chromosomes for normal follicular development was determined in the 1960s. A critical region on the X chromosome (POF1), which ranges from Xq13 to Xq26, which relates to normal ovarian function has been identified, as has a second gene of paternal origin (POF2), which is located at Xq13.3–q21.1. Idiopathic POF can be familial or sporadic, and the familial pattern of inheritance is compatible with X-linked (with incomplete penetrance) or an autosomal dominant mode of inheritance. In Turner syndrome, complete absence of one X chromosome (45XO) results in ovarian dysgenesis and primary ovarian failure. Familial POF has been linked with fragile X permutations. Fragile X mutations occur at least 10 times more often in women with POF than the general population. Women with Down's syndrome (Trisomy 21) also have an early menopause. The BEPS syndrome is a rare autosomal dominant condition that leads to congenital abnormalities of the eye, including blepharophimosis, ptosis and epicanthus inversis. In BEPS I, eyelid malformation cosegregates with POF and has been mapped to chromosome 3q.17.

Follicle-stimulating hormone receptor gene polymorphism and inhibin B mutation

Resistance to the action of gonadotrophins can lead to the clinical features of POF, and this has been shown in a cohort of Finnish families. This is a very rare cause. In addition, a mutation in the inhibin gene (see Chapter 1) that has a frequency 10-fold higher than in control patients (7% versus 0.7%) has been identified. These patients experienced ovarian failure at an early age – often before the second decade of life.

Enzyme deficiencies

A number of enzyme deficiencies have been found to be associated with an increased risk of POF. The most common of these is the autosomal recessive condition of galactosaemia, in which there is a deficiency in the enzyme galactose-1-phosphate uridyltransferase. Accumulation of galactose results in damage to the liver, eyes and kidneys. The risk of POF has been found to be as high as 81% in affected females, and the cause seems to be a galactose-induced reduction in total germ-cell development during oogenesis. Other proposed mechanisms include accelerated follicular atresia and biologically inactive isoforms of follicle-stimulating hormone (FSH). Other enzyme abnormalities associated with POF include deficiencies of 17α-hydroxylase, 17–20 desmolase and cholesterol desmolase. Deficiency of 17α-hydroxylase can prevent oestradiol synthesis, which leads to primary amenorrhoea and elevated levels of gonadotrophins, even though developing follicles are present.

Patients with a deficiency of cholesterol desmolase are not able to produce biologically active steroids and rarely survive to adulthood.

Autoimmune disease

Premature ovarian failure is frequently associated with autoimmune disorders, particularly hypothyroidism (25%), Addison's disease (3%) and diabetes mellitus (2.5%). Other co-existing conditions may include Crohn's disease, vitiligo, pernicious anaemia, systemic lupus erythematosus or rheumatoid arthritis. Addison's disease may be present as part of a polyglandular failure syndrome. The type I syndrome, which is associated with adrenal failure, hypoparathyroidism and chronic mucocutaneous candidiasis and occurs mainly in children, is associated with POF. The type II syndrome may present much later with hypothyroidism and is less consistently associated with POF.

The prevalence of antibodies directed against the ovary has been the subject of significant research. Circulating anti-ovarian antibodies have been found in 10–69% of women with POF but also in a significant number of controls. Anti-gonadotrophin receptor antibodies have been isolated, but their significance remains unclear. Antibodies directed against steroid-producing cells have proved most promising in terms of predicting which patients may develop ovarian failure as part of the polyglandular syndrome; however, these women constitute a minority of those with POF.

Secondary premature ovarian failure

Secondary POF is becoming more important as survival after the treatment of malignancy continues to improve. However the development of techniques to conserve ovarian tissue or oocytes before therapy is instigated should help with maintenance of fertility. The causes of secondary POF are detailed below.

Chemotherapy and radiotherapy

The likelihood of ovarian failure after chemotherapy or radiotherapy depends on the agent used, dosage levels, interval between treatments and, particularly, the age of the patient, which probably reflects the age-related progressive natural decline in the oocyte pool. The prepubertal ovary is relatively resistant to the effects of chemotherapeutic alkylating agents. Attempts to suppress the ovarian activity of women of reproductive age with oral contraceptives or gonadotrophin hormone-releasing analogues in order to mimic this protection have produced conflicting results.

Radiation-induced ovarian failure usually results in sterility when the total dose exceeds 6 Gy. As with chemotherapy, however, prepubertal girls are more resistant to irradiation. Normal menstruation after treatment does not necessarily mean the ovaries are unaffected, and premature menopause can occur, resulting in a shorter reproductive span. Surgical transposition of the ovaries outside of the direct field of treatment has been described. A successful term pregnancy also depends on a normal uterine environment that is not only receptive to implantation but also able to accommodate normal growth of the fetus. The degree of damage to the uterus depends on the total dose of radiation and the site of irradiation. The prepubertal uterus is more vulnerable to the effects of pelvic irradiation, with doses of radiation of 14–30 Gy likely to result in uterine dysfunction. High-dose pelvic radiotherapy in young women will have long-term effects on the uterine vasculature and development. Adverse pregnancy outcomes have been described for women treated with total body irradiation and include an increased risk of early pregnancy loss, preterm birth and delivery of infants with low or very low birthweights. An excess risk of infants of low birthweight and preterm birth also exists among mothers who received abdominal irradiation for Wilms' tumour in childhood.

Bilateral oophorectomy or surgical menopause

This results in an immediate menopause, which may be intensely symptomatic. The implications of this procedure require detailed discussion with the patient in view of the increased morbidity and mortality in those who cannot, or will not, take oestrogen replacement.

Hysterectomy without oophorectomy

This can induce ovarian failure in the immediate postoperative period, where in some cases it may be temporary, or at a later stage, where it may occur sooner than the time of natural menopause. This is an area of controversy and may depend on ovarian function preceding hysterectomy. The diagnosis may be difficult, as not all women have acute symptoms, and in the absence of a uterus, the pointer of amenorrhoea is absent. A case could be made for annual estimates of levels of FSH in women who have had a hysterectomy before the age of 40 years.

Infection

Tuberculosis and mumps are infections that have been implicated most commonly. The increasing incidence of tuberculosis and the emergence of multi-drug resistant strains of bacilli is of concern. In most cases, normal ovarian function returns after infection with mumps. Malaria, varicella and shigella infections have also been implicated in POF.

Presentation and assessment

The most common presentation is secondary amenorrhoea or oligomenorrhoea in a woman younger than 40 years, which may not necessarily be accompanied by hot flushes. Use of combined oestrogen and progestogen or long-acting depot contraceptives results in a proportion of women who present with persistent amenorrhoea when these forms of contraception are stopped.

Co-existing disease must be detected, particularly hypothyroidism, Addison's disease, diabetes mellitus and any chromosome abnormalities in women with primary ovarian failure – especially those who have not achieved successful pregnancy (see Box 11.1 and Chapter 5). The diagnostic usefulness of ovarian biopsy outside the context of a research setting has yet to be proved.

Box 11.2

Investigation of premature menopause

- Estimates of levels of follicle-stimulating hormone in serum (×2)
- Thyroid function tests
- Autoimmune screen for polyendocrinopathy
- Chromosome analysis, especially in women younger than 30 years
- Estimates of bone mineral density through dual X-ray absorptiometry (DXA) (optional)
- Adrenocorticotrophic hormone stimulation test if Addison's disease is suspected (optional)

Consequences of oestrogen deficiency

Women with untreated premature menopause are at increased risk of developing osteoporosis and cardiovascular disease but at lower risk of breast malignancy (Box 11.2). Mean life expectancy in women with menopause before the age of 40 years is 2.0 years shorter than that in women with menopause after the age of 55 years. Premature menopause can lead to reduced peak bone mass (if the women is younger than 25 years) or early bone loss thereafter. The increased risk of coronary heart disease has been noted especially in smokers.

Management

Counselling

Patients must be provided with adequate information. Women may find it a difficult diagnosis to accept, especially if they wish to have children. National self-support groups for POF exist, such as the Daisy Network in the UK (http://www.daisynetwork.org.uk/), and these provide helpful psychological support for many women. Women need to be aware that ovulation may occur again, often intermittently, and cyclical menstrual bleeding or even pregnancy can result.

Hormone replacement therapy

Oestrogen replacement therapy is the mainstay of treatment for women with POF and is recommended until the average age of natural menopause (52 years in the UK, see Chapter 1). This view is endorsed by regulatory bodies such as the Committee on Safety of Medicines in the UK. No evidence shows that oestrogen replacement increases the risk of breast cancer to a level greater than that found in normally menstruating women, and women with POF do not need to start mammographic screening early. Hormone replacement therapy (HRT) or the combined oestrogen and progestogen contraceptive pill may be used. No clinical trial evidence attests the efficacy or safety of the use of non-oestrogen-based treatments, such as bisphosphonates, strontium ranelate or raloxifene, in these women (see Chapter 8).

A commonly adopted form of treatment is the combined oral contraceptive pill. The latter has the psychological benefit of being a treatment used by many of the patient's peer group. There is a paucity of controlled trial data on how to base treatment decisions. The only direct comparison of ethinyloestradiol and conjugated equine oestrogen is a study of 17 women with Turner syndrome. In this short study, no difference was seen between the two oestrogens with respect to effect on the endometrium, hyperinsulinaemia or lipid profile. Ethinyloestradiol had a more potent effect on markers of bone turnover and suppression of gonadotrophins. Women with POF who take HRT may need a higher dose of oestrogen to control vasomotor symptoms than women in their 50s.

Some patients report persistent tiredness, lack of energy, reduced libido or sexual function despite apparently adequate doses of oestrogen replacement. This may be more common in oophorectomized women, and consideration should be given to additional treatment with testosterone. Testosterone implants may be provided along with subdermal oestrogen, if this form of replacement has been chosen (see Chapter 6). If testosterone patches and gels presently undergoing clinical trials, are licensed for use in women, they may provide an alternative.

Fertility issues

The lifetime chance of spontaneous conception in women with karyotypically normal POF has been estimated at 5–15%, with the age of the patient at the time of diagnosis being an important determinant. Assessment of ovarian reserve is a controversial area. Parameters of ovarian reserve that have been studied include FSH, luteinizing hormone (LH), oestradiol, inhibin B, anti-Mullerian hormone, total antral follicle count and ovarian volume. As yet, no single clinically useful test is available to predict ovarian reserve accurately, and a combination of markers may ultimately be more helpful

Donor oocyte in vitro fertilization (IVF) is the treatment of choice for women with primary and secondary POF. Women with spontaneous, karyotypically normal POF have similar success rates to women who undergo conventional IVF. Patients can be reassured that there is no urgency for treatment after a diagnosis of POF. The age of the oocyte rather than the age of the recipient determines the chance of success. The use of a sibling's oocyte may decrease the likelihood of pregnancy.

Oocyte donation is also an option for women with Turner syndrome, and pregnancy rates in observational studies are similar to those with oocyte donation for other indications. The risk of miscarriage, however, is greater. Cardiovascular and other complications, such as hypertension and pre-eclampsia, occur more frequently in women with Turner syndrome. It has been suggested that embryo transfer be limited to a single embryo to avoid additional complications as a result of multiple pregnancies. Pretreatment screening to detect previously undiagnosed maternal congenital cardiac abnormalities is essential.

Very few options are available for preventative therapy before radiotherapy and chemotherapy. Mature oocytes and ovarian tissue cannot be cryopreserved easily; however, successful pregnancies have been achieved. The collection of mature oocytes requires ovarian stimulation, which may not be advisable in women with oestrogen-dependent malignancies. In addition, these techniques are not suitable for prepubertal patients. Cryopreservation of embryos may be possible before treatment – if time allows and fertility drugs are not contraindicated.

Further reading

Aetiology

Aittomaki K, Lucena JLD, Pakarinen P, et al. Mutation in the follicle-stimulating hormone receptor gene causes hereditary hypergonadotrophic ovarian failure. Cell 1996;82:959–68.

Amati P, Gasparini P, Zlotogora J, et al. A gene for premature ovarian failure associated with eyelid malformation maps to chromosome 3q22-q23. Am J Hum Gen 1996;58:1089–92.

Conway GS, Payne NN, Webb J, et al. Fragile X permutation screening in women with premature ovarian failure. Hum Reprod 1998;13:1184–7.

Farquhar CM, Sadler L, Harvey SA, Stewart AW. The association of hysterectomy and menopause: a prospective cohort study. BJOG 2005;112:956–62.

Groff AA, Covington SN, Halverson LR, et al. Assessing the emotional needs of women with spontaneous premature ovarian failure. Fertil Steril 2005;83:1734–41.

Hoek A, Schoemaker J, Drexhage HA. Premature ovarian failure and ovarian autoimmunity. Endocr Rev 1997;18:107–34.

Howell S, Shalet S. Gonadal damage from chemotherapy and radiotherapy. Endocrinol Metab Clin North Am 1998;27:927–43.

Pal L, Santoro N. Premature ovarian failure (POF): discordance between somatic and reproductive aging. Ageing Res Rev 2002;1:413–23.

Raven P, Lind C, Nilas L. Lack of influence of simple premenopausal hysterectomy on bone mass and bone metabolism. Am J Obstet Gynecol 1995;172:891–5.

Shelling AN, Burton KA, Chand AL, et al. Inhibin: a candidate gene for premature ovarian failure. Hum Reprod 2000;15:2644–9.

Siddle N, Sarrel P, Whitehead M. The effect of hysterectomy on the age at ovarian failure: identification of a subgroup of women with premature loss of ovarian function and literature review. Fertil Steril 1987;47:94–100.

Watson NR, Studd JW, Garnett T, et al. Bone loss after hysterectomy with ovarian conservation. Obstet Gynecol 1995;86:72–7.

Wallace WH, Thomson AB, Saran F, Kelsey TW. Predicting age of ovarian failure after radiation to a field that includes the ovaries. Int J Radiat Oncol Biol Phys 2005;62:738–44.

Consequences of premature menopause

Hu FB, Grodstein F, Hennekens CH, et al. Age at natural menopause and risk of cardiovascular disease. Arch Intern Med 1999;159:1061–6.

Jacobsen BK, Knutsen SF, Fraser GE. Age at natural menopause and total mortality and mortality from ischemic heart disease: the Adventist Health Study. J Clin Epidemiol 1999;52:303–7.

Ossewaarde ME, Bots ML, Verbeek AL, et al. Age at menopause, cause-specific mortality and total life expectancy. Epidemiology 2005;16:556–62.

Titus-Ernstoff L, Longnecker MP, Newcomb PA, et al. Menstrual factors in relation to breast cancer risk. Cancer Epidemiol Biomarkers Prev 1998;7:783–9.

Management

Beerendonk CC, Braat DD. Present and future options for the preservation of fertility in female adolescents with cancer. Endocr Dev 2005;8:166–75.

Donnez J, Dolmans MM, Demylle D, et al. Livebirth after orthotopic transplantation of cryopreserved ovarian tissue. Lancet 2004;364:1405–10.

Guttman H, Weiner Z, Nikolski E, et al. Choosing an oestrogen replacement therapy in young adult women with Turner syndrome. Clin Endocrinol 2001;54:159–64.

Lutchman Singh K, Davies M, Chatterjee R. Fertility in female cancer survivors: pathophysiology, preservation and the role of ovarian reserve testing. Hum Reprod Update 2005;11:69–89.

National Collaborating Centre for Women's and Children's Health. Fertility: Assessment and Treatment for People with Fertility Problems. London: RCOG Press, 2004:126–7.

Nelson LM, Covington SN, Rebar RW. An update: spontaneous premature ovarian failure is not an early menopause. Fertil Steril 2005;83:1327–32.

Revel A, Elami A, Bor A, et al. Whole sheep ovary cryopreservation and transplantation. Fertil Steril 2004;82:1714–15.

Shifren J, Braunstein GD, Simon JA, et al. Transdermal testosterone treatment in women with impaired sexual function after oophorectomy. N Engl J Med 2000;343:682–8.

Silber SJ, Lenahan KM, Levine DJ, et al. Ovarian transplantation between monozygotic twins discordant for premature ovarian failure. N Engl J Med 2005;353:58–63.

Sung L, Bustillo M, Mukherjee T, et al. Sisters of women with premature ovarian failure may not be ideal ovum donors. Fertil Steril 1997;67:912–16.

Tucker D. Premature ovarian failure. In: Rees M, Hope S, Ravnikar V, eds. The Abnormal Menstrual Cycle. Abingdon: Taylor and Francis, 2005:111–22.

12 Women with a co-existent medical condition

Pelvic disorders
Breast disorders
Cardiovascular disease
Endocrine disease
Neurological disease
Gastrointestinal conditions
Autoimmune disease
Other
Further reading

In the presence of some pre-existing medical conditions, a more careful assessment of the patient is indicated and modification of treatment may be advisable. Health professionals may prefer to refer such patients to a specialist clinic to explore oestrogen and non-oestrogen-based options. Different types and routes of oestrogen-based treatments are discussed. Chapter 8 discusses treatments not based on oestrogen. The following conditions may require special evaluation.

Pelvic disorders

Fibroids

Fibroids (leiomyomas) are oestrogen-dependent tumours that tend to shrink after the menopause. These may become enlarged with oestrogen treatment and cause heavy or painful withdrawal bleeds, so the patient should be advised of this. The evidence of the effect of different types of hormone replacement therapy (HRT), including tibolone, on fibroid growth is poor. Ultrasound examinations may be helpful in documenting the fibroids, and, if clinically indicated, regular pelvic examinations are recommended. Limited data suggest that raloxifene shrinks fibroids.

Endometriosis

This condition can present a difficult management problem, as oestrogen treatment can theoretically reactivate the disease, even when the patient has had apparent surgical removal of all the endometriotic tissue. Concerns are disease recurrence and malignant changes arising from the presence of residual endometriosis. The risks, however, seem to be small, and the evidence base of various strategies is poor. Patients with a history of endometriosis may be at particular risk of the long-term consequences of oestrogen deficiency as a consequence of repeated courses of gonadotrophin hormone-releasing analogues or bilateral oophorectomy. Some gynaecologists avoid starting oestrogen-based HRT for the first six months after oophorectomy, preferring to give a progestogen alone, continuous combined therapy or tibolone to control vasomotor symptoms when the patient has extensive disease. No good evidence base is available on whether to recommend an unopposed regimen, an opposed continuous combined regimen or tibolone. Management of potential recurrence is best monitored by responding to the recurrence of symptoms. No data exist with regard to raloxifene.

Cervical and ovarian cancer and cervical dysplasia

These are not oestrogen-dependent conditions, and oestrogen replacement is not contraindicated. Some doubt exists, however, with regard to endometrioid ovarian cancer, and progestogen addition may be recommended. The use of HRT does not seem to influence adversely the risk of ovarian cancer in women who carry BRCA mutations.

Endometrial cancer

Unopposed oestrogen therapy in non-hysterectomized women is associated with an increased risk of endometrial hyperplasia and cancer. As a consequence prior endometrial carcinoma is often listed in datasheets as an absolute contraindication to oestrogen-replacement therapy; however, no data show an increased risk of recurrence or mortality. On the contrary, a reduction in frequency of relapses is shown, together with longer disease-free intervals and survival times. Furthermore, no advantage of addition of progestogen has been shown, but the numbers of patients were small. A systematic review concluded that there seems to be no indication for adjuvant progestogens after early stage endometrial cancer. Progestogens, however, do play a role in patients with advanced or recurrent disease. Evidence with regard to tibolone or raloxifene is scant.

Breast disorders

Family history of breast cancer

Little evidence shows that the use of HRT in patients with a family history of breast cancer will further increase their risk, but, for the most part, studies have failed to accurately document family history. No evidence supports the safety of herbal medicines in these women. Any woman with a significant family history should be referred to a specialist breast clinic to determine her personal risk, without which informed decisions cannot be made (see Chapter 5).

Benign breast disease

Benign breast disease encompasses a diverse range of conditions – not all of which are associated with an increased risk of breast cancer. Of these changes, only those of ductal or lobular atypical hyperplasia are associated with a significant increase in risk. Although HRT may be associated with mastalgia and promotion of breast cysts, no convincing evidence shows that the risk of breast cancer is increased in patients with benign disease. Failure to accurately categorize benign disease, however, prevents determination of whether or not women involved in these studies were at a significantly increased risk of breast cancer.

Previous breast cancer

Survivors of breast cancer with menopausal symptoms pose a management problem, as conventional advice is to avoid the use of exogenous oestrogens. Concerns also exist that survivors of breast cancer are at increased risk of osteoporotic fracture. Most clinical studies of patients with breast cancer who have been prescribed systemic HRT have not shown an adverse effect on survival; however, these involved small numbers of patients, with short-term follow-up. Early interim analysis of two randomized trials in Scandinavia (HABITS and Stockholm studies) have shown contradictory results. The increased risk of recurrence reported in HABITS has been suggested to be explained by the fact that most women randomized to HRT did not use concurrent tamoxifen and most used continuous combined HRT, whereas in the Stockholm study, most women took tamoxifen and had long-cycle combined HRT. The adverse results of the HABITS study, although based on a very small number of clinical events, resulted in the premature cessation of the Stockholm study (in which no increase in risk was found). It also halted the National UK randomized trial of HRT in symptomatic women with early-stage breast cancer. Currently, the effect of HRT is uncertain, and it is important to appreciate problems that arise from overinterpretation of preliminary outcomes – whatever effect is shown. The randomized LIBERATE trial of tibolone in survivors of breast cancer is continuing.

Low-dose vaginal oestrogens are not contraindicated for women with vaginal symptoms (see Chapter 6). For the moment, patients with breast cancer who have severe menopausal symptoms or in whom concerns exist about osteoporosis require guidance from the local oncology or specialist menopause clinic.

Cardiovascular disease

Hypertension

No evidence shows that oestradiol-based HRT increases blood pressure or has an adverse effect in women with hypertension. Rarely, conjugated equine oestrogens may cause severe hypertension that returns to normal when treatment is stopped. Data from trials of tibolone and raloxifene do not show an adverse effect on blood pressure.

Valvular heart disease

Hormone replacement therapy is not contraindicated in women with valvular heart disease. Women who take anticoagulants may have more problems with irregular or heavy bleeding, which requires an adjustment of the dose of progestogen relative to that of the oestrogen. Endometrial biopsy, if required, should be performed under antibiotic cover.

Hyperlipidaemia

In women, the most significant lipids are high-density lipoprotein cholesterol (HDL-C), triglyceride and lipoprotein(a). The increased risk associated with increased levels of triglycerides and low-density lipoprotein cholesterol (LDL-C) can be offset by increased levels of HDL. In terms of lipids, the ideal HRT would increase HDL-C without increasing triglyceride and decrease LDL-C and lipoprotein(a). The effects depend on the type of steroid and the route of administration. Oral oestrogen reduces lipoprotein(a) and LDL-C and increases HDL-C and triglycerides. The transdermal route is less effective at reducing lipoprotein(a) and LDL-C but does not increase triglycerides or HDL-C. The type of progestogen is also important. Oral HRT with a non-androgenic progestogen will increase HDL-C and triglycerides and decrease LDL-C and lipoprotein(a). Oral HRT with a 19-nortestosterone derivative will decrease LDL-C and lipoprotein(a) but will not increase HDL and will be neutral for triglycerides. Thus, HRT in these women needs to be tailored to their lipid profile: for example, in women with hypertriglyceridaemia, the transdermal route is preferred to the oral route (Table 12.1). Hormone replacement therapy can be combined with statins.

Raloxifene and tamoxifen reduce levels of total cholesterol and LDL-C while remaining neutral towards triglyceride and HDL-C. Although much discussed, as yet, no randomized controlled trial evidence is available for selective oestrogen receptor modulators for cardiovascular events. A large

Table 12.1

Effects of hormones on lipids

Hormone	Lipid			
	HDL	LDL	Triglyceride	Lipoprotein (a)
Ideal HRT	↑↑	↓↓	↓↓	↓↓
Oral oestrogen	↑	↓↓	↑	↓↓
Transdermal oestrogen	–	↓	↓	↓
Oral non-androgenic progestogen	↑	↓	↑	↓
Oral 19-nortestosterone progestogen	–	↓	↓	↓
Tibolone	↓	↓	↓↓	↓
Raloxifene	–	↓	–	↓

↑ Small increase
↓ Small decrease
↑↑ Big increase
↓↓ Large decrease
– No effect

randomized controlled trial of the effects of raloxifene on cardiovascular endpoints is currently underway (RUTH study). Similarly, no data exist for tibolone.

Venous thromboembolism

When taking the history, it is essential to assess the family history, the severity of any personal event and whether or not it was confirmed objectively. It can be difficult to know if a history of venous thromboembolism (VTE) – sometimes more than 20 years earlier – was a confirmed episode. When in doubt, if a patient was anticoagulated at the time, it is prudent to consider the event confirmed.

Women with a personal history of thrombosis

A history of VTE is the biggest risk factor for future VTE and is a relative contraindication to HRT. After a single episode of VTE, a constant risk of recurrence of 5% per year exists when anticoagulation is discontinued.

After careful consideration and discussion with the patient, however, it might be felt in some cases that the risk is outweighed by the benefits of HRT. A thrombophilia screen may then be justified, as the finding of a severe defect or a combination of defects might alter the perceived risk–benefit assessment. A negative thrombophilia screen must not be used to give false reassurance. The woman may be at high risk even though no pathological explanation is present. Women older than 50 years with a history of VTE within the previous year, in addition to thrombophilia screening, should be screened for underlying disease, including malignancy and connective tissue disorders. If a decision to use HRT is made, limited evidence suggests that the transdermal route might be safer. Occasionally, it is suggested that a woman is anticoagulated to allow HRT to be given. It has to be appreciated that about one in 400 patients on warfarin bleed to death each year, so this is rarely the best option. As raloxifene and progestogens in doses higher than those used for contraceptive purposes increase the risk of VTE, these are probably best avoided (see Chapter 8). No data are available for tibolone in this situation.

Women with a family history of thrombosis
To test women with a family history of thrombosis for hereditary thrombophilia is only fully informative if a family study is performed. Without a family study, a negative screen must not be used to give false reassurance, as these women may still be at increased risk. For example, if a first-degree relative has a significant thrombotic history but a negative thrombophilia screen, testing cannot offer any reassurance. Women found to have antithrombin deficiency or combined defects have the greatest risk. If a decision to use HRT is made, limited evidence suggests that the transdermal route might be safer. The comments made above regarding raloxifene, progestogens and tibolone are relevant here.

Women with a personal history of thrombosis on long-term warfarin
Hormone replacement therapy, raloxifene, progestogens and tibolone can be prescribed in these women, as the risk of recurrence should be very small provided anticoagulation continues.

Hormone replacement therapy and surgery
If HRT is stopped, the increased risk of VTE disappears rapidly, so HRT could be stopped four weeks before elective surgery. A more practical alternative is to continue HRT and ensure that adequate prophylaxis is given against VTE.

Endocrine disease
Diabetes mellitus
Diabetes mellitus is the most common chronic disease in the industrialized world. In North America and Europe, the prevalence in adults is 7–8%, and more than 100 million cases are estimated worldwide. Type 2, or non-insulin dependent diabetes mellitus (NIDDM), accounts for 90% of all cases. It affects both men and women in equal frequency and is most common in obese people older than 40 years. Hormone replacement therapy seems to decrease the

incidence of type 2 diabetes mellitus, as well as improving glycaemic control, with results varying according to the type and route of administration. It also improves lipid profiles, and transdermal delivery seems to decrease triglyceride levels in particular. Data on the effect of HRT on coronary heart disease (CHD) are conflicting; however, it might be beneficial in younger postmenopausal diabetic women, whereas it cannot be advised for women older than 60 years with, or at high risk of, cardiovascular disease. Cardioprotective adjunctive treatments (such as statins or low-dose aspirin) may be advised in diabetic women with risk factors for CHD and can be prescribed concomitantly with HRT. However, HRT is currently not recommended solely for the possible prevention of cardiovascular disease. Osteoporosis is reported as a potential complication of type 1 diabetes mellitus, but the effects of type 2 diabetes mellitus on bone mass are conflicting. As type 1 and 2 diabetes increase the risk of endometrial cancer, women with these conditions must receive a progestogen if the uterus is intact.

Thyroid disease

Thyroid disease is common and affects women more than men. A large population study has found that the prevalences of previously diagnosed hyperthyroidism are 2.5% in women and 0.6% in men, of hypothyroidism are 4.8% and 0.9% and of goitre are 2.9% and 0.4%, respectively. A past history of hyperthyroidism of any aetiology is associated with an increased risk of osteoporosis and hip fracture, particularly in postmenopausal women. This may result from endogenous overproduction or over-replacement of thyroxine in women with hypothyroidism or those who receive thyroid-stimulating hormone (TSH)-suppressing thyroid hormone treatment for thyroid cancer. In contrast, the risk to bone seems to be minimal in women with primary hypothyroidism treated with thyroid hormone replacement without suppression of TSH. Patients who present with hyperthyroidism should be screened for osteoporosis. Thyroxine replacement should be adjusted so that TSH is not suppressed. Thyroid replacement is not a contraindication for HRT, but the dose of thyroxine may need to be increased because oestrogen can increase concentrations of thyroxine-binding globulin. Conversely, the dose of thyroid replacement may need to be reduced when HRT is stopped.

Neurological disease

Migraine

This condition is more common in women than men and is usually a condition of the reproductive years, starting during the teens and 20s. It is unusual for migraines to start after the age of 50 years. Menstruation is often a significant trigger, and the menopause marks a time of increased migraine. Hormone replacement therapy can help – not only by stabilizing fluctuations in oestrogen that are associated with migraine but also by relieving night sweats that disturb sleep. No good evidence supports the idea that HRT aggravates migraine. As migraine can be triggered by fluctuating concentrations of oestrogen, the transdermal route is favoured over the oral route, because it produces more stable levels of oestrogen. Too high an oestrogen dose can trigger migraine aura, which usually resolves as the dose is reduced. Unlike the contraceptive pill, no data suggest that the risk of ischaemic stroke is increased in women with migraine with aura who take HRT. Sequential progestogen treatment may be a trigger for migraine. The strategies that can be used are changing the type of progestogen (19-nortestosterone to 17-hydroxyprogesterone derivatives), changing to continuous combined therapy and delivering the progestogen transdermally or into the uterus with the levonorgestrel device (see Chapter 6). Hormone replacement therapy is not contraindicated by treatments for migraine such as triptans.

Epilepsy

Data about the menopause, HRT and epilepsy are limited. The number of patients is small, and the type and dose of HRT have not been examined systematically. Of concern is that some antiepileptics are inducers of liver enzymes, and herbal preparations used for menopausal symptoms may interact with them (see Chapter 10). No data as yet confirm whether the transdermal route is preferable to the oral route. Whether women who take oral therapy should take an increased dose (extrapolating from combined oral contraceptive usage) is not yet known. Furthermore, data show that anticonvulsant treatments cause changes in the metabolism of calcium and bone and may lead to decreased bone mass with the risk of osteoporotic fractures. Widely used antiepileptic drugs, such as phenytoin, carbamazepine and sodium valproate, are recognized to affect metabolism of vitamin D and to have direct effects on bone cells that lead to impaired bone mass.

Parkinson's disease

Epidemiological studies associate the postmenopausal use of oestrogen with a reduction in the risk of Parkinson's disease. In animal models, oestrogens have been shown to attenuate neuronal death in rodent models of Parkinson's disease. The evidence regarding acute effects of HRT and Parkinson's disease again is limited. Transdermal delivery of 17β-oestradiol seems to display a slight prodopaminergic (that is, antiparkinsonian effect) without consistently altering dyskinesias. It would seem, therefore, that the use of HRT is not contraindicated.

Gastrointestinal conditions

Gallbladder disease

In the UK, about 8% of the population older than 40 years has gallstones; this figure increases to more than 20% in people older than 60 years. Randomized trials (HERS and WHI) have shown an increased risk of gallbladder disease with oral HRT (see Chapter 7). The non-oral route is usually recommended in women with a pre-existing disease, but little evidence supports this.

Liver disease

A non-oral route of oestrogen treatment is advised in women with liver disease to avoid the first liver pass, but the evidence is limited. Some types of liver disease, such as primary biliary cirrhosis, are associated with osteoporosis. A specialist opinion should be obtained.

Crohn's disease

A major consideration in women with Crohn's disease is the increased risk of osteoporosis, which may result from the disease itself or the long-term use of corticosteroids. The transdermal route of HRT is usually preferred to ensure adequate absorption.

Coeliac disease

Bone mineral density is decreased in women with coeliac disease, with about 47% of women on a gluten-free diet having osteoporosis. The mechanism that underlies osteoporosis in women with coeliac disease is likely to be related to calcium malabsorption, which leads to increased parathyroid hormone secretion, which, in turn, increases bone turnover and cortical bone loss. Malabsorption of vitamin D is probably of less importance. Again, the transdermal route for oestrogen delivery may be preferred for women in whom HRT is indicated.

Autoimmune disease

Rheumatoid arthritis

This is a systemic disorder that manifests itself primarily as a chronic, inflammatory polyarthropathy. It is six times more common in the sixth decade than in the second decade, and women are affected about 2.5 times more frequently than men. Women with rheumatoid arthritis are at increased risk of osteoporosis, and this may be related to disease severity, steroid use and immobility caused by the disease. Furthermore, bone resorption is increased in women with rheumatoid arthritis, and this is related to disease activity. The use of oestrogen or non-oestrogen-based treatments will depend on the woman's symptoms, bone mineral density and preference. No evidence shows that the use of HRT affects the risk of developing rheumatoid arthritis, and it does not induce flares in menopausal women. Bisphosphonates are also effective at reducing the risk of fracture.

Systemic lupus erythmatosus

Systemic lupus erythematosus (SLE) is a rare multi-system rheumatic disease characterized by fever, arthritis, pleuropericarditis, skin rashes, grand mal seizures, kidney failure or pancytopenia. It characteristically flares during pregnancy. The increased life expectancy of patients with SLE means that early cardiovascular mortality and glucocorticoid-associated bone loss are now important issues. Surveys have found that fractures occur in 12.3% of patients with SLE. The occurrence of fractures in women with SLE is now five-fold higher than that in normal women from the American population. Older age at diagnosis of SLE and longer use of corticosteroids are associated with time from diagnosis of SLE to fracture.

In women with SLE and a previous VTE or those positive for lupus anticoagulant, HRT should be considered with caution. Concerns exist that oestrogen may increase flares, but evidence is sparse.

Other

Asthma

In women who have used systemic steroids, bone mineral density needs to be assessed (see Chapter 5). There seems to be a small increase in the risk of asthma and asthma-like symptoms in women who use HRT. The use of HRT, however, does not seem to worsen pre-existing asthma. No evidence exists with regard to tibolone or raloxifene.

Otosclerosis

This condition is inherited as a Mendelian dominant characteristic and leads to progressive deafness. Evidence suggests that pregnancy can aggravate this condition, and it can rarely worsen with oral contraceptives. No data, however, show that HRT causes a deterioration of the disease. As the natural course of the disease is progressive, it is likely that hearing will become more impaired in women who use HRT in the long term.

Malignant melanoma

This is a controversial area. It is generally accepted that no association exists between the risk of melanoma and the use of HRT. Reports about a relation between the prognosis of melanoma and HRT are contradictory. Oestrogen receptors are present on melanomas, but it seems unlikely that oestradiol has a direct effect on melanogenesis.

Lentigo maligna is the precursor of lentigo maligna melanoma. It is most common in the eighth decade, is found on the cheek or neck and correlates closely with exposure to ultraviolet radiation. That lentigo maligna possesses both oestrogen and progesterone receptors suggests a possible role of these steroids in malignant transformation.

After transplantation

Bone mass is reduced in a high percentage of patients after organ or marrow transplantation, with the prevalence of osteopenia or osteoporosis reported to be as high as 80%. Up to 65% of transplant recipients will experience an osteoporosis-related fracture, and the likelihood of developing such a serious outcome is dependent on pre-existing disease and immunosuppressive therapy. Post-transplant glucocorticoid therapy is thought to play a major role in the further reduction in bone mass seen in these patients. The additional role of other immunosuppressant treatments in bone loss is less clear, but some evidence suggests that cyclosporin A and tacrolimus (FK506) produce osteopenia as a result of high bone turnover. Anti-osteoporotic strategies need to be considered.

Renal failure

Patients with end-stage renal disease (ESRD) are at increased risk for early menopause, osteoporosis, cognitive dysfunction and cardiovascular disease. Data are needed in this population to define the benefits of oestrogen and non-oestrogen-based treatments.

Further reading

Pelvic disorders

Fedele L, Bianchi S, Raffaelli R, Zanconato G. A randomized study of the effects of tibolone and transdermal estrogen replacement therapy in postmenopausal women with uterine myomas. Eur J Obstet Gynecol Reprod Biol 2000;88:91–4.

Kotsopoulos J, Lubinski J, Neuhausen SL, et al. Hormone replacement therapy and the risk of ovarian cancer in BRCA1 and BRCA2 mutation carriers. Gynecol Oncol 2005;[Epub ahead of print].

Martin-Hirsch PL, Jarvis G, Kitchener H, Lilford R. Progestogens for endometrial cancer. Cochrane Database Syst Rev 2000:(2)CD001040.

Matorras R, Elorriaga MA, Pijoan JI, et al. Recurrence of endometriosis in women with bilateral adnexectomy (with or without total hysterectomy) who received hormone replacement therapy. Fertil Steril 2002;77:303–8.

Mueck AO, Seeger H. Hormone therapy after endometrial cancer. J Br Menopause Soc 2003;9:161–5.

Palomba S, Orio F Jr, Russo T, et al. Antiproliferative and proapoptotic effects of raloxifene on uterine leiomyomas in postmenopausal women. Fertil Steril 2005; 84:154–61.

Ramirez PT, Frumovitz M, Bodurka DC, et al. Hormonal therapy for the management of grade 1 endometrial adenocarcinoma: a literature review. Gynecol Oncol 2004; 95:133–8.

Sagsveen M, Farmer JE, Prentice A, Breeze A. Gonadotrophin-releasing hormone analogues for endometriosis: bone mineral density. Cochrane Database Syst Rev 2003;(4):CD001297.

Soliman NF, Evans AJ. Malignancy arising in residual endometriosis following hysterectomy and hormone replacement therapy. J Br Menopause Soc 2004; 10:123–4.

Suriano KA, McHale M, McLaren CE, et al. Estrogen replacement therapy in endometrial cancer patients: a matched control study. Obstet Gynecol 2001; 97:555–60.

Surrey ES, Hornstein MD. Prolonged GnRH agonist and add-back therapy for symptomatic endometriosis: long-term follow-up. Obstet Gynecol 2002;99:709–19.

Yang CH, Lee JN, Hsu SC, et al. Effect of hormone replacement therapy on uterine fibroids in postmenopausal women – a 3-year study. Maturitas 2002;43:35–9.

Zupi E, Marconi D, Sbracia M, et al. Add-back therapy in the treatment of endometriosis-associated pain. Fertil Steril 2004;82:1303–8.

Breast disorders

Chen Z, Maricic M, Bassford TL, et al. Fracture risk among breast cancer survivors: results from the Women's Health Initiative Observational Study. Arch Intern Med 2005;165:552–8.

Col NF, Hirota LK, Orr RK, et al. Hormone replacement therapy after breast cancer: a systematic review and quantitative assessment of risk. J Clin Oncol 2001; 19:2357–63.

Dupont WD, Page DL, Parl FF, et al. Estrogen replacement therapy in women with a history of proliferative breast disease. Cancer 1999;85:1277–83

Fowble B, Hanlon AL, Patchefsky A, et al. The presence of proliferative breast disease with atypia does not significantly influence outcome in early-stage invasive breast cancer treated with conservative surgery and radiation. Int J Radiat Oncol Biol Phys 1998;42:105–15.

Hartmann LC, Sellers TA, Frost MH, et al. Benign breast disease and the risk of breast cancer. N Engl J Med 2005;353:229–37.

Holmberg L, Anderson H. HABITS (hormonal replacement therapy after breast cancer – is it safe?), a randomised comparison: trial stopped. Lancet 2004; 363:453–5.

Kroiss R, Fentiman IS, Helmond FA, et al. The effect of tibolone in postmenopausal women receiving tamoxifen after surgery for breast cancer: a randomised, double-blind, placebo-controlled trial. BJOG 2005;112:228–33.

Meurer LN, Lena S. Cancer recurrence and mortality in women using hormone replacement therapy: meta-analysis. J Fam Pract 2002;51:1056–62.

O'Meara ES, Rossing MA, Daling JR, et al. Hormone replacement therapy after a diagnosis of breast cancer in relation to recurrence and mortality. J Natl Cancer Inst 2001;93:754–61.

Rohan TE, Miller AB. Hormone replacement therapy and risk of benign proliferative epithelial disorders of the breast. Eur J Cancer Prev 1999;8:123–30.

Santen RJ, Mansel R. Benign breast disorders. N Engl J Med 2005;353:275–85.

von Schoultz E, Rutqvist LE. Menopausal hormone therapy after breast cancer: the Stockholm randomized trial. J Natl Cancer Inst 2005;97:533–5.

Cardiovascular disease

Anderson GL, Limacher M, Assaf AR, et al. Effects of conjugated equine estrogen in postmenopausal women with hysterectomy: the Women's Health Initiative randomized controlled trial. JAMA 2004;291:1701–12.

Cagnacci A, Baldassari F, Arangino S, et al. Administration of tibolone decreases 24 h heart rate but not blood pressure of post-menopausal women. Maturitas 2004;48:155–60.

Cushman M, Kuller LH, Prentice R, et al. Estrogen plus progestin and risk of venous thrombosis. JAMA 2004;292:1573–80.

de Valk-de Roo GW, Stehouwer CD, Meijer P, et al. Both raloxifene and estrogen reduce major cardiovascular risk factors in healthy postmenopausal women: a 2-year, placebo-controlled study. Arterioscler Thromb Vasc Biol 1999;19:2993–3000.

Grady D, Wenger NK, Herrington D, et al. Postmenopausal hormone therapy increases risk for venous thromboembolic disease. The Heart and Estrogen/progestin Replacement Study. Ann Intern Med 2000;132:689–96.

Herrington DM, Vittinghoff E, Howard TD, et al. Factor V Leiden, hormone replacement therapy, and risk of venous thromboembolic events in women with coronary disease. Arterioscler Thromb Vasc Biol 2002;22:1012–17.

Karalis I, Beevers G, Beevers M, Lip G. Hormone replacement therapy and arterial blood pressure in postmenopausal women with hypertension. Blood Press 2005; 14:38–44.

Keeling DM. Hormone replacement therapy, thrombosis and thrombophilia. J Br Menopause Soc 2005;11:74–5.

Rossouw JE, Anderson GL, Prentice RL, et al. Risks and benefits of estrogen plus progestin in healthy postmenopausal women: principal results from the Women's Health Initiative randomized controlled trial. JAMA 2002;288:321–33.

Royal College of Obstetricians and Gynaecologists. Hormone Replacement Therapy and Venous Thromboembolism. Guideline 19. London: Royal College of Obstetricians and Gynaecologists, 2004.

Stevenson JC. Metabolic effects of hormone replacement therapy. J Br Menopause Soc 2004;10:157–61.

Endocrine disease

Anderson KE, Anderson E, Mink PJ, et al. Diabetes and endometrial cancer in the Iowa women's health study. Cancer Epidemiol Biomarkers Prev 2001;10:611–16.

Arafah BM. Increased need for thyroxine in women with hypothyroidism during estrogen therapy. N Engl J Med 2001;344:1743–9.

Bjoro T, Holmen J, Kruger O, et al. Prevalence of thyroid disease, thyroid dysfunction and thyroid peroxidase antibodies in a large, unselected population. The Health Study of Nord-Trondelag (HUNT). Eur J Endocrinol 2000;143:639–47.

Cummings SR, Nevitt MC, Browner WS, et al. Risk factors for hip fracture in white women. Study of Osteoporotic Fractures Research Group. N Engl J Med 1995;332:767–73.

Eaton SE, Webster J, Allahabadia A. Thyroid disease and the menopausal woman. J Br Menopause Soc 2003;9:82–4.

Ferrara A, Quesenberry CP, Karter AJ, et al. Current use of unopposed estrogen and estrogen plus progestin and the risk of acute myocardial infarction among women with diabetes: the Northern California Kaiser Permanente Diabetes Registry, 1995-1998. Circulation 2003;107:43–8.

Greenspan SL, Greenspan FS. The effect of thyroid hormone on skeletal integrity. Ann Intern Med 1999;130:750–8.

Hippisley-Cox J, Pringle M, Crown N, Coupland C. A case-control study on the effect of hormone replacement therapy on ischaemic heart disease. Br J Gen Pract 2003;53:191–6.

Kanaya A, Herrington D, Vittinghoff E, et al. Glycaemic effects of postmenopausal hormone therapy: the Heart and Estrogen/progestin Replacement Study. Ann Intern Med 2003;138:1–9.

Khoo CL, Perera M. Diabetes and the menopause. J Br Menopause Soc 2005;11:6–11.

Margolis KL, Bonds DE, Rodabough RJ, et al. Effect of oestrogen plus progestin on the incidence of diabetes in postmenopausal women: results from the Women's Health Initiative Hormone Trial. Diabetologia 2004;47:1175–87.

Nicodemus KK, Folsom AR. Type 1 and type 2 diabetes and incident hip fractures in postmenopausal women. Diabetes Care 2001;24:1192–7.

Rossi R, Origliani G, Modena M. Transdermal 17β estradiol and risk of developing type 2 diabetes in a population of healthy, non obese postmenopausal women. Diabetes Care 2004;27:645-9.

Zendehdel K, Nyren O, Ostenson CG, et al. Cancer incidence in patients with type 1 diabetes mellitus: a population-based cohort study in Sweden. J Natl Cancer Inst 2003;95:1797-800.

Neurological disease

Abbasi F, Krumholz A, Kittner SJ, Langenberg P. Effects of menopause on seizures in women with epilepsy. Epilepsia 1999;40:205–10.

Bousser MG, Conard J, Kittner S, et al. Recommendations on the risk of ischaemic stroke associated with use of combined oral contraceptives and hormone replacement therapy in women with migraine. The International Headache Socie'

Task Force on Combined Oral Contraceptives & Hormone Replacement Therapy. Cephalalgia 2000;20:155–6.

Currie LJ, Harrison MB, Trugman JM, et al. Postmenopausal estrogen use affects risk for Parkinson disease. Arch Neurol 2004;61:886–8.

Green PS, Simpkins JW. Neuroprotective effects of estrogens: potential mechanisms of action. Int J Dev Neurosci 2000;18:347–58.

Harden CL, Pulver MC, Ravdin L, Jacobs AR. The effect of menopause and perimenopause on the course of epilepsy. Epilepsia 1999;40:1402–7.

Koppel BS, Harden CL, Nikolov BG, Labar DR. An analysis of lifetime fractures in women with epilepsy. Acta Neurol Scand 2005;111:225–8.

MacGregor EA. Menstrual migraine. In: Rees M, Hope S, Ravnikar V, eds. The Abnormal Menstrual Cycle. Abingdon: Taylor and Francis, 2005:197–218.

Pack AM, Morrell MJ, Marcus R, et al. Bone mass and turnover in women with epilepsy on antiepileptic drug monotherapy. Ann Neurol 2005;57:252–7.

Rosciszewska D. Menopause in women and its effects on women. Neurol Neurochir Polska 1986;12:315–19.

Gastrointestinal conditions

Cirillo DJ, Wallace RB, Rodabough RJ, et al. Effect of estrogen therapy on gallbladder disease. JAMA 2005;293:330–9.

Clements D, Compston JE, Evans WD, Rhodes J. Hormone replacement therapy prevents bone loss in patients with inflammatory bowel disease. Gut 1993;34:1543–6.

Hulley S, Grady D, Bush T, et al. Randomized trial of estrogen plus progestin for secondary prevention of coronary heart disease in postmenopausal women. Heart and Estrogen/progestin Replacement Study (HERS) Research Group. JAMA 1998;280:605–13.

Johnson CD. ABC of the upper gastrointestinal tract: upper abdominal pain: gallbladder. BMJ 2001;323:1170–3.

Ormarsdottir S, Mallmin H, Naessen T, et al. An open, randomized, controlled study of transdermal hormone replacement therapy on the rate of bone loss in primary biliary cirrhosis. J Intern Med 2004;256:63–9.

Scott EM, Gaywood I, Scott BB. Guidelines for osteoporosis in coeliac disease and inflammatory bowel disease. British Society of Gastroenterology. Gut 2000;46(Suppl 1):I1–8.

Autoimmune disease

Buyon JP, Petri MA, Kim MY, et al. The effect of combined estrogen and progesterone hormone replacement therapy on disease activity in systemic lupus erythematosus: randomized trial. Ann Intern Med 2005;142:953–62.

Daniels M, Huskisson EC, Spector TD. A randomised controlled trial of the hormone replacement therapy on disease activity in postmenopausal arthritis. Ann Rheum Dis 1994;53:112–16.

vsen CE, Nelson JL, et al. Non-contraceptive hormones and the risk of rheumatoid arthritis in menopausal women. Int J Epidemiol 1994;23:1248–55.

Kreidstein S, Urowitz MB, Gladman DD, Gough J. Hormone replacement therapy in systemic lupus erythematosus. J Rheumatol 1997;24:2149–52.

Lange U, Illgner U, Teichmann J, Schleenbecker H. Skeletal benefit after one year of risedronate therapy in patients with rheumatoid arthritis and glucocorticoid-induced osteoporosis: a prospective study. Int J Clin Pharmacol Res 2004;24:33–8.

Lee C, Ramsey-Goldman R. Osteoporosis in systemic lupus erythematosus mechanisms. Rheum Dis Clin North Am 2005;31:363–85.

Lodder MC, de Jong Z, Kostense PJ, et al. Bone mineral density in patients with rheumatoid arthritis: relation between disease severity and low bone mineral density. Ann Rheum Dis 2004;63:1576–80.

Yee CS, Crabtree N, Skan J, et al. Prevalence and predictors of fragility fractures in systemic lupus erythematosus. Ann Rheum Dis 2005;64:111–13.

Other

Barr RG, Wentowski CC, Grodstein F, et al. Prospective study of postmenopausal hormone use and newly diagnosed asthma and chronic obstructive pulmonary disease. Arch Intern Med 2004;164:379–86.

Kramer HM, Curhan GC, Singh A. Permanent cessation of menses and postmenopausal hormone use in dialysis-dependent women: the HELP study. Am J Kidney Dis 2003;41:643–50.

Naldi L, Altieri A, Imberti GL, et al. Cutaneous malignant melanoma in women. Phenotypic characteristics, sun exposure, and hormonal factors: a case-control study from Italy. Ann Epidemiol 2005;15:545–50.

Persson I, Yuen J, Bergkvist L, Schairer C. Cancer incidence and mortality in women receiving estrogen and estrogen-progestin replacement therapy – long-term follow-up of a Swedish cohort. Int J Cancer 1996;67:327–32.

Ramsey-Goldman R, Dunn JE, Dunlop DD, et al. Increased risk of fracture in patients receiving solid organ transplants. J Bone Miner Res 1999;14:456–63.

Shane E, Addesso V, Namerow PB, et al. Alendronate versus calcitriol for the prevention of bone loss after cardiac transplantation. N Engl J Med 2004;350:767–76.

Smith MA, Fine JA, Barnhill RL, Berwick M. Hormonal and reproductive influences and risk of melanoma in women. Int J Epidemiol 1998;27:751–7.

Thompson W. Otosclerosis and hormone replacement therapy: fact or fiction? J Br Menopause Soc 1999;5:54.

Troisi RJ, Speizer FE, Willett WC, et al. Menopause, postmenopausal estrogen preparations, and the risk of adult-onset asthma. A prospective cohort study. Am J Respir Crit Care Med 1995;152:1183–8.

Index

Page references to *figures, tables and boxes* are shown in *italics*